NCT Book of
First Foods

Other titles in this series:

Antenatal Tests
Postnatal Depression
Potty Training

NCT Book of
First Foods

Weaning guide with easy recipes

Ravinder Lilly

Thorsons
An Imprint of HarperCollins*Publishers*
in collaboration with National Childbirth Trust Publishing

Thorsons/National Childbirth Trust Publishing
Thorsons is an Imprint of HarperCollins*Publishers*
77–85 Fulham Palace Road
Hammersmith, London W6 8JB

Published by Thorsons and
National Childbirth Trust 1998
5 7 9 10 8 6

Ravinder Lilly asserts the moral right to
be identified as the author of this work

A catalogue record for this book
is available from the British Library

ISBN 0 7225 3603 8

Printed and bound in Great Britain by
Omnia Books Limited, Glasgow

'He who has health has hope, and he who has hope has everything.'

Arabian Proverb

Contents

Introduction: Eat Well Today for a
Healthy Tomorrow   ix

Part I   *The Right Start*   1
1   Nutrition Notes   3
2   Milk: The Only Food for Young Babies   14
3   What's Good for Babies   25
4   When to Wean   30
5   Your Older Infant (6 to 9 Months)   45
6   9 to 12 Months   54

Part II   *Recipes*   61
7   Guidelines Before You Begin   63
8   First Food Recipes   66
9   5 to 6 Months   75
10   6 to 9 Months   85
11   9 to 12 Months   122

       Useful Addresses   146
       Index   148

Introduction

Eat Well Today for a Healthy Tomorrow

Food is one of the greatest pleasures of life, but it is also essential for life itself. The type of food babies and children eat regularly can affect their chances of having good health and ill health, and is just as important as getting enough food. Certain degenerative conditions such as heart disease, tooth damage, obesity and high blood pressure in later life have been linked with a poor or restricted intake of nutrients in early life.

Right from first tastes, your baby will start to set the foundations for eating habits in later life. So, even at this very early stage, it is important to encourage your baby's interest in food and offer a healthy, varied diet.

What Makes a Diet Healthy?

The foods that experts recommend for adults today are very similar to those eaten by our distant ancestors. Once, much of our diet was composed of foods of vegetable origin: cereals, grains, pulses, vegetables and fruits. Meat, fish and poultry were eaten in smaller amounts.

These days there is no longer any need to hunt or forage for foods, and our supermarket shelves are laden with produce from all over the world, including many manufactured and processed foods that bear little resemblance to the original produce. Many more fatty, sugary and refined foods are available, but less marketing effort is made to encourage the appeal of vegetables, wholegrains and fruits. It seems that, although finding food has become much, much easier, actually eating well has become more difficult.

In fact a varied diet, with plenty of fresh whole foods, is all that is needed.

Eating healthily need not be dreary or difficult. You don't have to force yourself or your family to eat foods that you hate – choose from the huge variety of foods available and make up your own recipes. It needn't mean hard work, either – just make one small step at a time until you are all eating healthily. Remember – eat well today for a healthy tomorrow.

I

The Right Start

Nutrition Notes

All foods are made up of one or more of the seven nutritional 'building blocks': carbohydrates, proteins, fats, vitamins, minerals (including trace elements), water and fibre. No single food contains all the nutrients essential for good health, so a healthy diet has to contain all these 'building blocks' in the right proportions.

The Macronutrients: Proteins, Carbohydrates and Fats

Proteins, carbohydrates and fats provide the energy (calories) in the diet. Calories are the fuel needed to fire body processes, much as petrol in a car provides the engine with the fuel it needs. If more calories are taken than are used, the spare energy is converted to fat and stored.

Proteins

Proteins are essential for the building and repair of cells and tissue. Proteins are themselves made up of smaller building blocks called amino acids.

Both animal and vegetable foods can supply protein. Proteins from animal foods (such as dairy produce and meat) provide all of the essential amino acids, while those of vegetable origin (cereals and grains) tend to be low in one or more essential amino acids. Mixing different types of non-meat proteins (like rice and pulses or bread and lentils) improves the quality of the protein intake and helps to ensure all the amino acids are obtained in the right proportions. Most people in the UK get enough protein in their diet, but vegans and vegetarians need to be careful that they are eating a good mix of vegetable foods.

Animal Sources of Protein

❑ meat
❑ fish
❑ poultry
❑ eggs
❑ dairy products like milk, cheese and yoghurt

Non-meat Sources

❑ grains such as wheat, rice, millet and oats, and foods made from them like bread products and pasta

- soya beans and products made from them like tofu
- nuts and nut butters
- seeds
- lentils (red and green, for example)
- pulses such as red kidney beans and black–eye beans
- bread and bread products

These foods tend to be less expensive than animal sources of protein and are lower in fat.

Breastmilk is an excellent source of protein.

Carbohydrates

Carbohydrates may be divided into starchy or simple according to their chemical make-up.

The starchy (complex) carbohydrates in foods like potatoes, rice, pasta, bread and cereals are a good source of fibre, and can be a rich source of vitamins and minerals.

The simple (refined) carbohydrates such as sugar are often termed 'empty calories' as they provide calories but no other nutrients.

Humans have a natural liking for sweetness, which perhaps evolved as a type of natural defence mechanism: a fruit that is ripe and good to eat tastes sweet, while a food which is past its best, like milk which has gone off, tastes sour.

Today, refined sugar is cheap and freely available and is added to many manufactured foods. Eating many high-sugar foods frequently will cause dental decay and experts recommend that sugary foods and drinks should be limited. Babies under one year old should not have sugar added to foods or drinks.

Fat

Fat provides the insulation material for our bodies, protects internal organs, and helps keep tissue healthy. Women tend to have more body fat than men and this is related to their reproductive function: fat is naturally laid down in pregnancy to provide the concentrated energy resources needed while breastfeeding. Fat is an essential nutrient, but most adults eat too much.

Fat provides the most concentrated source of energy; in other words, it provides a lot of calories in a small volume. Because of this, it is a very important nutrient for babies and young children who have high requirements for calories but small stomachs. It is also an important source of fat-soluble vitamins A and D, and indeed these vitamins would not be absorbed at all without fat. Babies and toddlers should *not* be given a low-fat diet.

Breastmilk and formula milk supply energy because they are high in fats, so it is important to offer either breast- or formula milk for at least the first year. Even after one year, your baby should drink full-fat cow's milk. If your toddler enjoys a mixed diet, semi-skimmed milk can be taken after two years, but skimmed milk should not be offered until your child is five years old.

Depending on their chemical make-up, fats are classified as saturated or unsaturated. There are three types:

1 Saturated fats: These tend to be of animal origin (the exceptions are coconut and palm oil) and are usually solid at room temperature. Eating too much saturated fat has been linked with raised blood cholesterol and an increased risk of heart disease. Saturated fat is found in meat and meat products; dairy produce like cheese, butter, milk and cream, and in lard, suet and dripping. Experts recommend that this type of fat should be reduced in the diet.

2 Polyunsaturated fats: These usually come from vegetable or fish sources and are usually liquid at room temperature. They can help to lower blood cholesterol and nutritionists recommend that some saturated fat should be replaced with the polyunsaturated oils found in nuts and seeds like sunflower, corn, and safflower.
3 Monounsaturated fats don't raise cholesterol levels and may even help to lower them. Food sources of monounsaturated oils include olive oil and avocados.

The body cannot make certain fats, which must be supplied by the diet. The best sources of these essential fats are plant oils such as corn, rapeseed and sunflower. The oils from oily fish such as mackerel, herring, salmon, and pilchard supply another type of polyunsaturated fat which research has shown to be beneficial to health.

Fibre or NSP

Fibre is the name given to a range of vegetable substances which are essential to health even though they cannot be digested by humans. Naturally fibrous foods are bulky, and swell in the stomach, helping to speed up the passage of foods through your body and so preventing gut disorders like constipation. Fibre also encourages chewing and healthy gums. Fluids must be taken with fibre, or constipation could be made worse. Recently, fibre has been renamed non-starch polysaccharide (NSP).

Do Babies Need NSP?

Babies have small tummies but a very high need for nutrients. Fibre dilutes calories and is bulky, so a diet high in fibre is filling and leaves little room for other foods. This is why a high-fibre diet is not recommended for children under five years old. But don't exclude it altogether. Fibre helps to exercise the bowels, so you should introduce some in infancy, in the form of fruits, vegetables and oats.

Water

About two-thirds of human body weight is made up of water. It is an essential part of all body cells.

Breastfed babies do not need extra water, even in hot climates. If your baby is bottlefed, you may want to offer cooled, boiled water on warm days. And, once you have started to introduce a mixed diet, try offering a drink of cooled, boiled water or well-diluted fruit juice (diluted 50:50 with water) to quench thirst.

Vitamins Explained

Even though they are required in only small amounts by the body, vitamins are essential for most body processes. They cannot be manufactured by the body (except vitamin D, which is made by the action of sunlight on the skin) and need to be taken in the diet. Luckily they are found in a wide variety of foods. There are two types: fat-soluble and water-soluble. The fat-soluble vitamins (A, D, E and K) can be stored in the body. The water-soluble vitamins (B group and C) need to be taken in the diet daily and are easily destroyed by cooking.

Antioxidants

Colourful vegetables and fruit – apricots, mangoes and carrots for example – contain antioxidant pigments like beta carotene. Their natural function is to help stop fats going rancid. They also help to mop up free radicals (rapidly moving molecules which can damage cells) and may help prevent degenerative conditions such as certain cancers.

The Functions of Vitamins and Where to Find Them

Vitamin	Function	Food sources
Vitamin A	Needed for healthy tissue and good eyesight, aids growth and resistance to infection. The body can convert the pigment beta carotene (which is found in highly coloured vegetables and fruits) into a form of vitamin A.	Liver, dairy products, eggs, fortified margarine and oily fish. Beta carotene is found in orange, red and dark green vegetables and fruit such as apricots, cantaloupe melon, sweet potatoes and broccoli.
B_1 (Thiamin)/B_2 (Riboflavin)/B_3 (Niacin)/B_6 (Pyridoxine)/B_{12} (Cyanocobalamin)	A large group of vitamins needed to break down fats, proteins, and carbohydrates and for the correct functioning of the nervous system and production of healthy blood.	Wholegrain cereals, green vegetables, pulses, nuts, liver, meat, milk, yeast extract, eggs, dairy products and fortified breakfast cereals.

Folate (folic acid)	Needed for healthy blood, prevents neural tube defects (where the spinal cord does not develop normally) in babies before birth.	Fortified breakfast cereals and bread, green leafy vegetables, potatoes. Pregnant women, and women hoping to become pregnant, should take folic acid supplements as part of a healthy diet.
Vitamin C	Helps maintain healthy skin, blood vessels and gums and aids the absorption of iron.	Fruits and vegetables, especially citrus fruits, peppers, strawberries, blackcurrants and other berry fruits, guavas, tomatoes, cauliflower and broccoli.
Vitamin D	Works with calcium to maintain healthy bones and teeth.	Oily fish, liver, eggs, and fortified margarine. The majority of our vitamin D is made by the action of sunlight on the skin.
Vitamin E	An antioxidant that helps maintain healthy cell structure.	Vegetable oils, whole-grains, wheatgerm, soya, nuts and seeds.
Vitamin K	Blood clotting and wound healing. Can be made by gut bacteria in older babies, children and adults.	Alfalfa, soya beans, liver, egg yolks, green vegetables

Minerals Explained

Minerals are inorganic substances needed for a range of body processes. They are classed as major minerals or trace elements according to the relative amounts needed by the body. There are many minerals in our diet, including zinc, magnesium, manganese, selenium, iodine, and cobalt. However, the two most important are iron and calcium.

Iron is necessary for healthy blood and for mental and physical development. Iron deficiency is the most common nutritional deficiency seen in children. Babies and children need a lot of iron for rapid growth and development.

Calcium is essential for strong bones and teeth. A lack of calcium can result in porous bones and even osteoporosis in later life.

Minerals: Their Functions and Where to Find Them

Calcium	Healthy bones and teeth, muscle function and blood clotting.	Dairy products, fortified soya products, fish with soft bones (salmon and pilchard) fortified flours, hard water.
Iron	Vital for healthy blood and normal development.	Red meat, offal, nuts, pulses, egg yolk, dried fruits (especially apricots), wholemeal bread, fortified cereals, oily fish, cocoa.

Potassium	Works with sodium chloride to control water balance.	Found in a variety of foods including milk, cereals, fruit and vegetables.
Fluoride	In controlled amounts, strengthens tooth enamel (excess causes mottling) and bones.	Edible bones of fish, added to tap water in some areas (ask your dentist for advice), also added to some toothpastes.
Sodium chloride	Maintains body water balance and aids transmission of nerve impulses. A high intake has been linked with high blood pressure and salt should *not* be added to a baby's food.	Table salt, processed foods, cured and smoked foods, added to many manufactured foods.

Healthy Eating for Adults and Babies

You can encourage your baby and child to enjoy a variety of foods by setting a good example yourself.

Five Steps to a Healthier Diet for Adults

1 Enjoy plenty of starchy carbohydrate foods like bread, potatoes, rice and pasta, but don't add masses of fatty or creamy sauces or oils.

2 Eat more vegetables and fruit.

3 Cut down on fat by choosing the leanest cuts of meat, switching to skimmed or semi-skimmed milk, and replacing some of the meat in your diet with pulses.
4 Cut down on salt by eating less processed food and experimenting with other flavourings.
5 Don't eat too many sugary foods.

Milk: The Only Food for Young Babies

The Question of Milk

Breastmilk provides everything your baby needs for optimum growth and development for the first six months. Manufacturers of artificial and baby milks strive to make their milks as close as possible to human milk; although they may fall short in ways, most artificial milks are nutritionally adequate for the first four to six months of life.

Even after you start to introduce your baby to other foods, milk will remain an important part of his diet. If your baby is breastfed, occasional feeds of your milk will continue to offer him some protection against infections, well into his second year.

Breastmilk

Breastmilk is the perfect food. It is exclusively designed (and continually adjusted) to meet the changing needs of your individual baby. Your body is preparing to breastfeed from the very early weeks of pregnancy; breastfeeding is the natural conclusion of the physical and hormonal changes of pregnancy and childbirth. Whether or not you decide to breastfeed, your breasts will produce colostrum and your body will lay down stores of fat to fuel lactation.

Five reasons why breastmilk is best for your baby:

1 Breastmilk is the complete food for your baby. It supplies all the nutrients, including vitamins and minerals, which he requires in the exact amounts needed, from the first moments after birth until at least six months of age. No extras are needed; the unique combination of foremilk and hindmilk ensures that his thirst is quenched and his hunger satisfied.

2 Breastmilk is a dynamic food. It changes to meet your baby's needs. If your baby is born prematurely, your milk will be suitable for him at that point in his life; when he is five months old, your milk will be ideal for a baby of that age.

3 Breastmilk is unique. It contains hormones, growth-promoting factors and essential fatty acids – each item unique to humans and necessary to promote optimal development of the brain and nervous system of your human baby. Scientists are constantly finding out new and wonderful things about breastfeeding.

4 Breastmilk is custom-made for human babies. It is constantly produced, hygienically stored and always available. Breastmilk is designed for your baby's immature digestive tract; it is easily digested with little waste. Breastmilk, unlike artificial baby milks, does not contain large quantities of cow's milk proteins. A completely

breastfed baby is therefore less likely to develop allergic conditions such as asthma and eczema.

5 Breastmilk is protective. Your colostrum – the milk produced in the first days after birth – is especially rich in antibodies. Antibodies are special substances which actively fight bacteria and other infective agents. This protection continues for as long as you breastfeed, allowing precious time for your baby's own immune system to develop effectively. Breastmilk is also protective against many non-infective diseases, such as heart disease and childhood leukaemia and diabetes.

Your Diet While Breastfeeding

Lactation (the production of milk) is an incredibly efficient process requiring only a slight increase in your calorie requirement. Furthermore, during pregnancy your body gets ready for lactation by preparing a valuable store of energy – the extra fat which appears on your hips and tummy.

Be guided by your appetite. Try to eat a variety of nutritious foods and drink enough fluid to satisfy your thirst. Don't try to restrict your food intake or start a 'slimming' diet until breastfeeding is well established, at around six to eight weeks. Remember that although making milk is not tiring in itself, the 24-hour care of a new baby certainly is. Now may not be the time to 'go without' – rather a time to spoil yourself and enjoy life!

Calcium and Breastfeeding

Calcium is a naturally occurring mineral vital for healthy bone development. Your baby will get all the calcium she needs from your breastmilk. There is some evidence that women lose some of the mineral content from their own bones during lactation. This loss may be reduced if mothers pay attention to their calcium intake whilst breastfeeding; good dietary sources of calcium are suggested on page 11. Current research indicates that bone density is readily regained once lactation ceases and there is some evidence that breastfeeding actually protects against hip fractures in later life.

Why Breastfeeding Is Good for *You*

1 It is healthy. There is evidence that women who breastfeed have a lower risk of ovarian cancer and pre-menopausal breast cancer. Some women find that breastfeeding helps them to lose the extra weight accumulated during pregnancy.

2 It is inexpensive. A year's supply of artificial baby milk costs in excess of £500; bottles, teats and sterilizing equipment add to the cost. A breastfeeding mother needs only a couple of supportive and comfortable bras.

3 It is convenient. Breastmilk is instantly available – day or night, at home, out shopping, travelling. No special equipment is required, no advance preparation needed. Breastfeeding cannot be delegated; it gives you and your baby a close, cozy time together. Breastfeeding allows you to sit down and rest!

Practice Makes Perfect

Breastfeeding is a skill which has to be learned and practised. The best way to learn is by watching another mother and baby together – videos, books and classes are poor seconds! The best way to practise is with your own baby, in quietness and privacy. You may want to have an experienced midwife or another mother to guide you – or you may prefer to take the first steps alone with your baby and, perhaps, a supportive partner.

The first few days of breastfeeding can be tricky, as you and your baby recover from the birth. Be kind to yourself. Rest as much as you can. Make getting to know your baby a priority – and ask for help from your midwife or NCT breastfeeding counsellor if things do not feel quite right.

Surround yourself with people who feel positive about breastfeeding; your antenatal class group who are probably learning with you, sisters or friends who have happily breastfed their own babies. If in doubt, read back through any breastfeeding leaflets or books you may have. Ask questions until you get answers – but make your own decisions. *You* are the expert on *your* baby!

Breastfeeding and Working

It is possible to both breastfeed and work. Remember that the vast majority of the world's babies depend on breastmilk and most of their mothers have no choice but to work long and hard outside the home. Women manage according to their circumstances, although for some it is obviously easier than for others. Factors that help include:

❑ a skilled and dependable substitute carer for your child in your absence
❑ a society (or, at least, an employer) who believes in the importance of young children and their families.

How you organize your daily life will depend on your baby's age, the time you need to spend away from your baby and how much time you devote to expressing breastmilk. Options range from expressing your milk at intervals throughout your working day to ensure that your baby is fed only breastmilk, to breastfeeding just at night or at week-ends, using artificial milk at other times.

Do not let the prospect of returning to work complicate your ear-ly weeks of breastfeeding. When you feel the two of you have got the knack of breastfeeding – after two or three weeks, maybe – it is prob-ably a good idea to offer your baby a small quantity of expressed milk in a bottle, simply to get her used to taking her milk in this way. Otherwise, enjoy your time together and remind yourself that you are giving her an excellent start in life; a recent study showed that working mothers of breastfed babies are less likely to need time off work to care for sick children.

Don't forget that you can express breastmilk and freeze it for later. Ask your health visitor or breastfeeding counsellor if you want more information.

The way that others see breastfeeding can affect the outcome of breastfeeding, so if you don't have the support of close family, especial-ly your partner, you are unlikely to breastfeed. You may need to find other sources of support such as an NCT breastfeeding counsellor

Not Always Easy

Although breastfeeding really is best for baby and for mother, there can be problems, but this need not mean that you are on your own or that you are unique. Although breastfeeding is natural, it is a skill that needs to be learned by mother and baby together, and undoubt-edly, you will need support.

Where to get more advice and support:

- ❏ your breastfeeding counsellor
- ❏ talking with other mums, for example at your NCT group
- ❏ your own mother
- ❏ friends and relatives

- your midwife (up to 10 days after the birth of your baby)
- your health visitor (after 10 days)
- *Breastfeeding your baby* is a comprehensive book about breast-feeding from NCT Publishing.

Other Milks Explained

If you decide to bottlefeed your baby, your baby will still thrive. And, even if you do breastfeed your baby, you are likely to bottlefeed at some time.

Formula Milk

Suitable from birth, formula milk is based on cows' milk which has been modified to closely mimic breastmilk. Manufacturers are continually involved in research in order to improve the formulas so that they are in line with continued research into the content and benefits of breastmilk. Formula milks are based on one of two proteins, whey (which many bottlefed babies are given from birth) or casein (which may be more appropriate for older, hungrier babies as it is believed to be more satisfying).

Follow-on Milks

These contain more iron than formula milk and can be given after six months of age, or you can continue to give breast- or formula milk.

Added Ingredients

Some kinds of formula milk have added ingredients, such as long-chain fatty acids, beta carotene or nucleotides. It is not clear whether these are better for your baby in the long term. Ask your midwife or health visitor for more details.

Soya Milk

A few babies may need to be given soya-based formula milk if there is evidence of allergy or intolerance to substances found in regular formula milk. If it is necessary, it will be prescribed by your doctor.

Cow's Milk

Cow's milk should not be given as a main milk drink before the age of a year as it does not contain the right balance of nutrients needed by a young baby. Some experts suggest that it can be used to make up cereals, for example after six months, but others recommend waiting until the baby is a year old. All cow's milk should be pasteurized to prevent the risk of infection from milk-borne micro-organisms.

Another reason that milk should not be used as a main milk drink until one year is because cow's milk is low in iron. The iron stores a baby is born with are generally sufficient until about four to six months of age, so iron-rich foods should be offered at a time that coincides with depleting stores.

After a year, full-fat cow's milk should be offered: it contains more energy (calories) than reduced fat milks (semi-skimmed and skimmed) and fat soluble vitamins A and D (because these vitamins are dissolved in fat, they are skimmed off when the fat is skimmed away). If your toddler has a good appetite and is eating a variety of foods, semi-skimmed milk may be offered after two years of age, but faddy or 'average' eaters should continue with whole milk until they are about five years of age. Skimmed milk should not be given before five years of age as it is too low in calories and does not have enough of the fat soluble vitamins.

Your baby will still need several breastfeeds or about a pint (500 ml) of breast-, formula or follow-on milk daily until around a year old. After this, your toddler should be getting most of her nutrition from a mixed diet and will need about 350 ml milk daily (about two thirds of a pint), or two servings of dairy products like yoghurt, cheese, custard, milky puddings and fromage frais.

Goat's and Sheep's Milk

Goat's and sheep's milk are not suitable for babies under one year of age as they are poor in a number of nutrients.

Bottlefeeding, Hygiene and Sterilization

All your baby's feeding equipment should be kept scrupulously clean as a young baby is susceptible to upset tummies.

Washing and Sterilizing Feeding Equipment

It is important to ensure your hands are clean – not only will they be dealing with washing and changing nappies, your baby may also enjoy gnawing on them for comfort. It goes without saying that you should wash your hands after changing your baby, after using the toilet, before and after preparing food and feeds and after handling pets and changing bins.

You won't need to sterilize bowls, plates and utensils but do make sure they are washed thoroughly in hot soapy water and rinsed well and allowed to drip dry if possible. Dishwashers are hygienic as they use high temperatures to wash dishes.

Cleaning Baby Bottles

To clean your baby's bottles, use a bottle brush to thoroughly clean the inside and outside to remove all traces of milk. Use hot, soapy water. Rinse well under running water and run some water through the teats to ensure they are not blocked. Place bottles, teat, rings, etc. in the sterilizer.

Methods of Sterilization

Boiling

Immerse bottles and teats in boiling water in a covered pan for 10 minutes. Leave until cool and keep covered until needed.

Chemical

Feeding equipment is immersed in a plastic sterilizing unit with a lid that contains a chemical sterilizer (either tablets or liquid). Equipment should be rinsed with boiled cooled water before use.

Microwaving

Using a special microwave sterilizer, equipment can be sterilized quickly and efficiently using very high temperatures.

Steam Sterilizing

Involves a special sterilizing unit (much like a kettle) which uses moist heat to destroy harmful micro-organisms. No rinsing is necessary.

Making Up a Feed

Wash and dry your hands. Use a sterilized bottle, cap, teat and disc. Pour in the required amount of boiled, cooled water. Add the required number of scoops of milk powder (remember to level out the powder with the back of the knife). Place the disc on the neck of the bottle and screw on the cap with the teat tightly. Shake well to disperse the powder. You can make up a day's supply of bottles and store them in the fridge to save time. It is very important to always follow the instructions on the packet so that feeds are at the right concentration: not too watery or too concentrated.

Warming Feeds

To warm the milk, place in a bowl of warm water. Health professionals do not recommend the use of microwaves to warm feeds as the heating can be uneven and lead to hot spots. If you do use this method of heating, shake the bottle well and test the temperature carefully before feeding your baby.

Discard unused feed and never reheat a feed that has been started.

3

What's Good for Babies

What Babies Need

A baby needs a lot of energy and nutrient-rich foods but has only a small capacity for eating. So they should not eat the high-fibre, low-fat diet recommended for adults. As already pointed out, high-fibre foods are bulky and low in calories and can fill up a baby's tummy, leaving little room for other foods. Fat is a very important nutrient for babies. It is a concentrated source of calories and an important source of fat-soluble vitamins A and D, which aid brain development in babies. So while adults are urged to reduce their fat intake, this does not apply to children under five years of age.

What Babies Don't Need

Sugar

Babies have a natural liking for sweet-tasting foods, but experts agree that first foods should be free of or low in added sugars. Sugar should be used only sparingly after the first year. Consuming too much sugary food and drink too frequently can lead to tooth damage; if food is sticky, residue remains on teeth for longer and leads to growth of bacteria. Also, if your baby eats too much sugary food, he may feel full and refuse to eat other foods that are more nutritious. Bacteria produce plaque, a sticky acidic substance which damages teeth and gums. Never add sugar or sugary drinks to your baby's bottle or feeder, as bathing the teeth in a sugar-rich fluid for long periods can cause rampant tooth damage and decay. When looking for sugar in bought foods, look for these words: sucrose, glucose, fructose, honey, golden syrup, hydrolysed starch, invert sugar, glucose syrup, dextrose, maltose. Don't give your baby ready-made food or drinks that contain artificial sweeteners. Artificial sweeteners are not suitable for children under three years old. Also, don't give your baby honey until he is at least one year old, as there is a very small risk that it contains harmful bacteria.

Salt (Sodium Chloride)

The kidneys regulate the concentration of water in the body. A baby's immature kidneys cannot deal with large amounts of salt, so don't add it to your baby's foods. Salt can be found in a number of foods (like meat and vegetables, bread and cheese) and this will supply all your baby's needs. Also, preferences for salt can become established from very early on, so do avoid salt and salty foods. Eating too much salt may lead to high blood pressure in later life. Your baby is not likely to suffer a deficiency of salt but could suffer from an excess, in the present and in the future. When looking for salt in foods, look for the word 'sodium', and remember that 'hydrolysed vegetable protein' is high in salt. Try not to give your baby food with hidden salt, such as yeast extract, stock cubes, ham and bacon. Don't give your baby smoked or salted fish.

Raw or Soft Boiled Eggs

Eggs can be offered after six months as long as both the white and the yolk are solid. Raw or soft cooked eggs are not suitable because of the risk of salmonella infection.

Paté and Soft Ripened Cheese

Paté and ripened cheeses like Brie and Camembert should be avoided until after one year to avoid the low risk of listeria infection.

A High-fibre Diet

As already mentioned, high-fibre foods tend to be low in calories, bulky and filling. They are not suitable for babies, who need a lot of calories and nutrients, but have a limited capacity for food. However, you should introduce your baby to small amounts of fibre by giving her fruit and vegetables.

Spices

Hot or strong spices such as chilli are not suitable for young babies, but milder spices like cumin and coriander may be acceptable and, indeed, are introduced in diluted quantities to young babies in some cultures.

Nuts

Be very careful with nuts. Chopped and whole nuts are not recommended until your child is five years of age – being small and hard, there is a risk of choking if they are eaten. On top of that, there is a risk of allergic reactions to all nuts, not just peanuts.

Wheat, Oats, Barley, Rye

Don't give your baby wheat, oats, barley or rye until she is six months old. A tiny number of babies react badly to these foods, which contain gluten.

Fatty Foods

Some foods are difficult for your baby to digest well at first. Avoid pork and food that contains pork, such as sausages, bacon, ham and pork roll, and oily fish, such as mackerel or sardines.

Additives

Additives are substances added to manufactured foods. They include flavourings (which enhance flavours), colourings (which enhance or alter colour), preservatives (which prolong shelf-life), and bulking agents (which increase the volume of foods but not the calories or nutritional content). First foods and drinks should be free of additives. Always check the label if you want to avoid certain additives, or write to the manufacturer. And look out for 'monosodium glutamate' (MSG) on the label as this flavouring has been linked by some experts to hyperactivity in young children.

Tea

Tea contains tannins, which can bind with iron and other minerals and so reduce the amount that a baby or child can absorb from food. Tea (and coffee) also contains the stimulant caffeine and is not suitable for babies.

Carbonated Drinks and Adult Drinks

Some carbonated drinks and adult drinks contain large amounts of sugar, others contain unsuitable additives, so they should not be given to babies or growing children.

4

When to Wean

The First Days

During the first four to six months of life, breast- or formula milk will provide all the nutrients your baby needs for growth and development. After this time, though, your rapidly developing baby will need more calories, iron and vitamins than milk alone can provide, and this is the time to start introducing your baby to a mixed diet. Milk will still be an important part of your baby's diet, but as she starts to take more food, she will require less and less milk. Remember to avoid cow's milk until much later – about the twelve-month stage.

Introducing foods other than milk to your baby is a gradual process. It starts with smooth, runny purées, and is complete when your baby has learned how to bite and chew, is enjoying three meals a day, using a cup and spoon, and joining in with family meals.

Not Too Early

Before four to six months, the digestive system is not ready for anything other than breast- or formula milk, so it is best to wait (unless you are advised otherwise by your doctor). Most babies are not ready for mixed feeding before four months because they have not developed sufficient coordination and can't maintain the posture needed to swallow. Their kidneys and digestive system may not be mature enough to cope with a more diverse diet. They may be more vulnerable to allergy and some reports have linked the early introduction of foods with increased risk of respiratory illness and eczema. So don't offer first foods too early. In the beginning, the small amounts taken will only introduce different tastes and textures to your baby and a mixed diet won't satisfy hunger until later on when larger quantities are taken.

When Is Your Baby Ready for First Tastes?

Babies are individual and develop at different rates, but you may want to consider introducing first foods when:

❑ your baby does not seem satisfied with her usual milk feeds and starts to demand more feeds;
❑ your baby appears to be more restless and starts to wake in the night, especially if she has learned to sleep through;
❑ your baby shows an interest in your food;
❑ your baby can pick up small things and put them in her mouth.

Don't Leave It Too Late...

Most babies should start to take a mixed diet by six months of age. One reason is that the iron stores laid down by your baby before her birth will be getting low (milk is not a good source of iron) and so she needs to start getting iron from foods. Also, research has shown that leaving the introduction of a mixed diet until relatively late may make babies less receptive to new tastes, flavours and textures, and more likely to refuse foods.

What About Pre-term Babies?

Babies born before 38 weeks are considered pre-term and have a greater need for certain nutrients like iron and zinc (because these start to be stored in your baby's body in the last weeks of pregnancy). They may need supplementation according to medical advice.

Premature babies will be ready to start mixed feeding between four and six months after the expected due date. So, for example, if your baby was two months premature, she will be ready for mixed feeding at six to eight months of age. Your health visitor or GP will advise you.

Special Considerations

Some babies need to have special attention paid to their diet. This may be due either to an allergy or intolerance to a food or food product, or it may be due to a rare metabolic disorder which affects the way a particular substance is handled by the body. If so, a medical diagnosis will be made after specialized testing, and your doctor may prescribe medication or refer you to a dietitian. With a specialist knowledge of nutrition and health, a state-registered dietitian will advise you how to maximize the chances of your baby obtaining all the nutrients needed for normal growth and development, while avoiding any unsuitable foods and substances. The dietitian will be able to offer alternative foods to those that need to be avoided and advise on any special organizations that can help.

Coeliac Disease or Gluten Intolerance

Gluten is a protein found in wheat, barley, rye and oats. Although it is usually harmless, in people who are gluten intolerant it can damage the lining of the gut and so lead to poor absorption of nutrients. Symptoms include bloating and loose, bulky, fatty stools. Gluten intolerance can be temporary, occurring after gastroenteritis, or it can be lifelong, as is the case in coeliac disease. Treatment is by a gluten-free diet, which a state-registered dietitian will tell you about. A baby with coeliac disease can grow and develop normally as long as gluten is omitted. A number of gluten-free foods can be bought or prescribed. These may be identified by the symbol of an ear of wheat with a cross drawn over it. Many manufactured products contain gluten, so do contact the Coeliac Society for advice on which manufactured products are free of gluten (see useful addresses at the end of the book).

Phenylketonuria

Phenylketonuria is a condition that is caused by too much of an essential amino acid called phenylalanine. It occurs when the enzyme that breaks down phenylalanine in the liver is absent. Without this enzyme, phenylalanine may build up to dangerous levels, sometimes leading to brain damage and delayed learning.

Today, all newborn babies are screened soon after birth for phenylketonuria by using the Guthrie test. The test is done a few days after birth, when your baby has had several milk feeds. Milk contains phenylalanine and the test detects whether too much is being left in the blood. Babies with phenylketonuria will be prescribed special formula milk, and a dietitian will advise on the diet in infancy and beyond.

Food Intolerance and Food Allergy

Generally, a bad reaction to food is due to a food intolerance. A person is said to have an intolerance to a food or food substance if eating that food leads to adverse symptoms but the reaction does not involve the immune system. An allergy, on the other hand, involves the immune system and antibodies are released to fight off the presence of the food 'intruder'. Symptoms vary but may include bloating, diarrhoea, rashes, swollen lips, coughs and wheezing and a runny nose. Sometimes, though, symptoms can be life-threatening (for example, an allergy to peanuts may be very serious).

Testing for allergies in very young babies is not usual practice. However if you or your family has a history of allergy (such as asthma or eczema) seek the advice of your GP before introducing a mixed diet as your children have a greater risk of food intolerance. If there is a family history of allergy in your family, you may want to:

- breastfeed for as long as possible, keeping an eye on your own diet as allergies can be passed on through breastmilk;
- introduce new foods slowly, one at a time, so you can pinpoint whether there is any reaction to that particular food;
- ask your health visitor for more advice.

Peanuts

Allergy to peanuts is rare, but potentially life-threatening. So you may want to delay the introduction of foods containing peanuts (usually in the form of peanut butter) until your child is three years old, especially if anyone in your family has eczema or asthma, or if there is a history of severe food allergy in your family. Other nuts can also be highly allergenic, and remember never to give chopped or whole nuts to children under the age of five because of the risk of choking.

Foods which commonly cause adverse reactions include:

- wheat, rye, oats and barley
- eggs (especially the whites)
- sesame seeds and products made from them
- nuts (especially peanuts)
- food made with soya
- citrus fruits such as oranges and lemons
- cows' milk and food made from cows' milk, such as cheese, yoghurt and ready-made food containing lactose or whey casein
- fish (including shellfish).

Because they are so allergenic, it is best to delay the introduction of these foods until your baby is six months old.

If you or anyone in your family has an allergy to peanuts (which is rare) seek medical advice about introducing any peanut products (such as peanut butter).

Cow's Milk Allergy

For bottle-fed infants with an allergy to cow's milk protein, suitable soy-based formulae are available. Your GP will give you advice on the suitability of products.

If you suspect that your child is intolerant to a particular food, do contact your GP, who will be able to test for intolerance and can refer you and your baby to a specialist. It is very important not to restrict your child's diet by cutting out foods. Expert advice is needed to ensure that the diet is balanced and provides all the nutrients your baby needs to grow and develop normally.

Be reassured, though, that if there is no family history of allergy, there is no need to worry about food intolerance. And, even if your baby is intolerant to a particular food, she may grow out of the intolerance in time.

Hyperactivity

Children who are said to be hyperactive tend to have a great deal of energy, are difficult to control, and exhibit a range of behavioural problems. Some experts believe that hyperactivity is related to certain food products. The American allergist Dr Ben Feingold developed a specific diet which carefully controls the intake of the foods which are thought to be linked with specific behavioural problems.

If you feel that your child is affected by certain food substances, speak to your GP. She may refer you to a specialist dietitian who can advise you and your child and ensure the diet remains balanced.

Offering First Tastes: When and How

Try offering first tastes from the tip of a shallow plastic spoon or your clean finger. Do choose a quiet time when both of you are relaxed and your baby isn't tired, perhaps at midday. Offer first tastes in the middle of a milk feed. This way, she won't be so hungry that she gets frustrated at trying this new way of eating, nor so full that she is just not interested.

Don't Be Discouraged

Babies are born with a strong sucking reflex, but eating foods from a spoon needs to be learned. So do take things at your baby's pace and don't be discouraged if she does not like the idea of a particular food at first. Just try again in a day or two, or mix a food with one that your baby has enjoyed already.

If your baby is not well or is teething, she may not be interested in solid food. Feed her on just her usual milk for a little while.

What About Organic Foods?

Free-range and organic foods are considered by a growing number of people to be safer (as they are free of pesticide residues and other chemicals), healthier, and more ethically sound (taking into account methods of animal rearing). Recent food scares (including the salmonella in eggs story in 1988 and the link between eating beef and BSE and CJD), have made sales of free-range produce grow rapidly. But what does 'free range' actually mean? Poultry and meat are said to be free range if the living conditions of the animals concerned meet certain standards. The living conditions are checked regularly. Freedom foods are products from animals that have been checked by the RSPCA to ensure that they have been well treated. Organic food is produced without artificial chemicals, fertilizers, pesticides, or growth hormones; producers are also subject to rigid testing, in cluding soil testing some years before certification is allowed. If you would like more information about organic or free range food, see useful addresses at the end of the book (the Soil Association and the RSPCA).

Homemade Foods

Preparing home-cooked foods for your baby is often better nutritionally for your baby than using manufactured ones. Yet the convenience of bought baby foods is undeniable, especially when travelling or early on when small amounts are taken. Many mothers offer a combination of bought and home-cooked foods.

But, before you buy, check the label. Manufactured weaning foods (and drinks) should be free of additives but, according to a recent report by the Food Commission, over 50 per cent of more than 400 babyfoods tested (desserts *and* savouries) had sugars added. A total of 60 per cent of the foods analysed contained starches and gums or fillers (such as maltodextrin, which is similar to the glue on stamps and envelopes) to bulk out the ingredients without making them more nutritious.

When buying manufactured foods, do get into the habit of reading labels. It is the only way to avoid unwanted extras.

> Don't add solid food such as cereal to your baby's milk or drinks because of the risk of choking. Also, adding solids to a bottle does not teach your baby about different textures and tastes, or how to chew.

At this early stage of weaning, offer single foods so that if something does not agree with your baby, you will know what it was. After two to four weeks, you can start mixing foods that your baby has enjoyed, for example potato with carrot or baby rice with pear.

Continue to widen the variety of foods offered, but do keep pace with your baby's needs. By the end of the first stage, you may be offering two or three meals a day. Continue to offer a wide range of fruits and vegetables and gradually make purées thicker.

Your baby is now on the road to enjoying a lifetime of delicious, nutritious eating.

What Can You Give Your Baby Now?

Baby rice, smooth runny purée of starchy vegetables (potatoes, sweet potato, carrot and parsnip), puréed cooked fruit (apple or pear), and puréed (very ripe) banana.

Wait-until-later Foods

- ❑ Soft–cooked eggs
- ❑ Whole or chopped nuts
- ❑ Sugar
- ❑ Salt
- ❑ Patés and soft ripened cheeses
- ❑ Hot spices such as chilli
- ❑ Wheat–based foods

Weaning-at-a-glance Calendar:

Four Months

The amount of foods your baby will take will increase gradually, but from early days until around six months you can expect to offer anything from 1 to 6 teaspoons of food. Some babies will not be ready to try solids at four months. There is no rush. Be led by your baby's appetite and interest in foods.

On Waking

Breast or bottle feed

Breakfast

Baby rice mixed with your baby's usual milk, or baby rice with some puréed fruit (1 or 2 tsp)
Breast or bottle feed

Lunch

Breast or bottle feed

Tea

Breast or bottle feed

Evening

Breast or bottle feed

Don't Give

- ❏ Wheat or wheat products
- ❏ Citrus or berry fruits
- ❏ Eggs
- ❏ Soft ripened cheeses
- ❏ Nuts
- ❏ Salt
- ❏ Sugar
- ❏ Milk or drinks other than baby's usual milk or boiled cooled water
- ❏ Tea

Weaning-at-a-glance Calendar:

Four-and-a-half Months

On Waking

Breast or bottle feed

Breakfast

Baby rice mixed with your baby's usual milk, or baby rice with some
puréed fruit (1 or 2 tsp)
Breast or bottle feed

Lunch

1 or 2 tsp puréed vegetables or fruit
Breast or bottle feed

Tea

Breast or bottle feed

Evening

Breast or bottle feed

Don't Give

- ❑ Wheat and wheat products
- ❑ Citrus and berry fruits

- ❑ Eggs
- ❑ Soft ripened cheeses
- ❑ Nuts
- ❑ Salt
- ❑ Sugar
- ❑ Chilli or strong spices
- ❑ Milk or drinks other than baby's usual milk or boiled cooled water
- ❑ Tea

Weaning-at-a-glance Calendar:

Five to Six Months

On Waking

Breast or bottle feed

Breakfast

Baby rice made with milk or water and/or a little mashed banana or other fruit
Breast or bottle feed
Puréed chicken or meat or lentils with vegetables
Puréed fruit
Drink of boiled, cooled water or well–diluted juice (from a cup)

Mid–morning and mid–afternoon, your baby may want a milk drink, so don't reduce the amount of milk offered; this will gradually go down as your baby starts to take more foods at mealtimes.

Tea

Puréed fruit or vegetables
Breast or bottle feed

Before Bed

Breast or bottle feed

What You Can Give Now

❑ Drinks of boiled cooled water or, with meals, well–diluted unsweetened fruit juice from a cup

Don't Give

❑ Wheat and wheat products
❑ Citrus and berry fruits
❑ Eggs
❑ Soft ripened cheeses
❑ Nuts
❑ Salt
❑ Sugar
❑ Chilli or strong spices
❑ Tea

As your baby becomes accustomed to mixed feeding, you can expect
her to take anything from 6 to 12 teaspoons.

Note: Fruit juice should be diluted half and half with boiled cooled
water.

5

Your Older Infant (6 to 9 Months)

Solid Foundations

Between six and nine months, you will see many changes in your baby as she continues to grow and develop rapidly. She may be able to sit up unaided for a short while, hold a spoon, and place objects in her mouth. She may already have a few teeth.

The Need for Variety

Now is the time to widen the variety of foods you offer your baby. No one food contains all of the many nutrients needed for good health. Now your baby is used to first tastes, giving her a variety of foods is the healthiest and the tastiest way to set her on the road to a lifetime of nutritious eating. Try experimenting with unusual vegetables and fruit, like fragrant fresh mango, tangy Sharon fruit, and sweet paw paw. Buy a little to see what your baby enjoys or add some yoghurt, oatmeal, or custard to make more expensive produce go further.

More Lumps, Please!

As your baby cuts a tooth or two, you can begin to offer coarser purées and soft lumps as well as mashed foods (although even without teeth, the gums are amazingly efficient at mashing food). Tackling lumps requires more coordination than swallowing purées, although some babies seem to be amazingly coordinated and spit out lumps with great accuracy. If this happens, continue to offer foods with soft lumps or thicker purées from the tip of a shallow spoon so the food slides off easily. Try mixing puréed food with a little baby rice which is slippery and may help the food go down a little more easily, or add more liquid.

Encouraging Self-feeding

Encouraging independent feeding can be a messy business, so be prepared to equip yourself with a large plastic sheet under the highchair, or lay down newspapers and use a soft bib to protect your baby's clothes. Use one spoon yourself and let your baby hold another to encourage her to have a go. Alternatively, let your baby hold the spoon you are holding while you guide it into her mouth.

What Can You Give Now?

Having first offered your baby vegetables, fruit and rice, you can now give her a greater variety of foods. Try lentils, meat, chicken and fish (make sure all the bones have been removed), well-cooked pulses like kidney beans, fromage frais, and full-fat plain or Greek yoghurt.

Wheat-based foods like bread, pittas, chappatis, and breadsticks, and breakfast cereals like Weetabix can also be introduced very gradually from around nine months, but do check the labels as some products are very high in added sugars (the higher the ingredient appears on the label, the more of it there is in the product). Once your baby is used to purées, it may be easier to give the solids before the milk feed.

Vitamin Drops

Government experts recommend that all breastfed children between six months and five years should take vitamin drops as a nutritional safety net. They contain vitamins A, C and D, are suitable for all vegetarians, and can be bought from child health clinics. However, bottle-fed babies and babies and children who are good eaters probably don't need to take extra vitamins. For more information, speak to your health visitor.

Your Baby's Milk

Your baby should still be having several breastfeeds, or about a pint of formula a day. If your baby is bottle-fed, you could switch to a follow-on formula which contains more iron. It is still worth using expressed breastmilk or formula milk to make up purées.

Teething Tips

Teeth will usually start to emerge from about six months. The gums may look red and sore and you may be able to feel the tip of the emerging tooth. Offering lumpier foods will help your baby develop chewing skills. Harder finger-foods can help to ease the pain and discomfort of teething. Try sticks of peeled carrot, hard baked crusts of toast or peeled slices of pear and apple.

> Your baby can now start to enjoy finger-foods, foods that she can hold. Try pieces of fruit, cooked vegetables, cooked pasta shapes and breads. Never leave your baby alone when eating because of the risk of choking.

Not Yet

Your baby still does not need salt, sugar, fatty foods, undercooked eggs, soft ripened cheeses, nuts, or strong spices like chilli.

Getting Enough Iron

Your baby was born with stores of iron that will last about six months or so. After this time, it is important to offer your baby iron-rich foods. This essential mineral is needed for proper growth and development, and research shows that iron deficiency is the most common nutritional deficiency seen in children. Good sources of iron include:

- ❑ red meat such as beef, and offal such as liver and kidney
- ❑ chicken or turkey, especially the dark meat
- ❑ eggs (both white and yolk should be cooked until solid)
- ❑ beans (such as aduki, kidney and haricot) and lentils (dhal)
- ❑ breakfast cereals, which are often fortified with iron (check the label)
- ❑ leafy green vegetables like broccoli, spring greens and cauliflower
- ❑ dried fruit such as apricots and raisins
- ❑ fortified baby cereals.

Vitamin C helps the body to absorb more iron from foods, so give your baby lots of things to eat that contain vitamin C, like pieces of orange, tomato, or kiwi fruit.

Microwaves

Although using a microwave is quick and easy for heating your baby's meals, they may heat food unevenly. There may be hot and cold spots and foods can be hotter in the middle of the container than on the outside. If you do use this method of heating, always stir the food to help distribute the heat evenly and check the temperature before you start to feed your baby.

Vegetarian Babies

A meat-free diet can provide all the nutrients required for proper growth and development. But it is important to take care that the diet supplies all the nutrients that meat would otherwise supply, and your baby receives all that she needs for good health, growth and development. Meat and fish are good sources of protein, iron, vitamin B_{12} and zinc. So, where can you find a good source of these nutrients in a meat-free diet?

- ❏ Protein: Offer a wide variety of pulses, grains like rice, cereals, and pasta. Mixing grains and pulses in a meal (like red kidney bean casserole with rice, or pulses and lentils with cereals) helps to provide a better mix of proteins.
- ❏ Iron: Offer fortified breakfast cereals with your baby's usual milk or iron-fortified soya milk. Soya and eggs are good sources of iron, as are pulses like red kidney beans and chickpeas, vegetables including dark green leafy vegetables and broccoli, dried fruits

like apricots, fortified breakfast cereals, beans and lentils, dried fruit and fortified baby cereals and wholemeal bread. Try to offer a source of vitamin C with meals to increase iron absorption.

❑ Calcium: Offer foods like milk and dairy products, tofu, calcium-fortified soy milk, bread and pulses.

❑ Vitamin B$_{12}$: This vitamin is not found naturally in foods of plant origin (with the exception of alfalfa). Good sources include forti-fied breakfast cereals and yeast extract (which is salty, so only add a scrape to your baby's toast or bread). For more advice, speak to your GP or health visitor, who may advise a supplement.

A vegan diet (one that excludes all animal foods) may be bulky and may pose a problem for a young baby. Continued breastfeeding is especially important for vegan babies in order to supply protein, calcium and other nutrients. Ask your health visitor for more advice and contact the Vegan Society (address at end of book).

Eating a wide variety of foods should help to ensure a good intake of vitamins, but if you are concerned, talk to your health visitor, who may recommend children's vitamin drops. As already explained, vitamin B$_{12}$ is found only in foods of animal origin, so if you exclude eggs and dairy products from your baby's diet it is particularly important to talk to your health visitor.

Protect Your Baby's Teeth

There is a huge range of drinks on the market including bottled and tap water, fruit juices, herbal drinks, and soft drinks such as squash-es, colas and tea.

While 'baby drinks' have fewer additives than adult varieties, they may contain sugars which can contribute to dental caries. To quench thirst, it is best to offer milk and/or cooled, boiled tap water. Those waters labelled as 'natural mineral water' (which may have higher solute contents) and effervescent waters are not always suitable for infants, so take care.

However, fruit drinks which contain vitamin C may be useful in aiding iron absorption. If they are given to infants, they should only be given sparingly and then only at mealtimes. Taking too much may mean that the appetite for more nutrient-dense drinks and foods is spoiled. Try to offer these drinks in a cup or feeder rather than a bottle, from six or seven months.

If bottle-fed, your baby will still be taking milk from a bottle and it is important to protect the teeth as much as you can. Letting your baby suck drinks other than water from a bottle will bathe the front teeth or incisors. This allows bacteria in the mouth to work on the sugars in baby drinks and milk and to produce the acid which causes decay. Never give sweetened drinks or juice from a bottle and always hold your baby when giving a milk feed from the bottle. Try giving some drinks from a cup with two handles to help protect the teeth.

Cleaning Your Baby's Teeth

You can start to clean your baby's mouth even before the teeth appear by using a piece of soft gauze wrapped around your finger. Later, clean new teeth with a child's toothbrush and a pea-sized amount of a specially formulated child's toothpaste every morning and evening. Ask your dentist if the water in your area is fluoridated. If not, she may suggest a fluoride product.

Enjoying New Flavours

Encouraging your baby to enjoy many new flavours will help to make sure that your baby grows to enjoy her greens and reds and yellows!

Weaning-at-a-glance Calendar:

Six to Nine Months

On Waking

Breast or bottle feed

Breakfast

Baby rice or other baby breakfast cereal with milk or water and puréed fruit
Toast fingers
Breast or bottle feed

Note: You may want to give your baby a main meal either at lunchtime or at teatime, but towards the end of this stage it may be better to offer a cooked meal at teatime to help establish the family routine.

Lunch

Puréed or minced meat, chicken, pulses, lentils, fish, grated cheese or mashed baked beans with potato, rice or pasta and vegetables
Stewed fruit or milk pudding
Drink of boiled, cooled water or diluted fruit juice from a cup

Tea

Toast fingers or bread and butter
Unsweetened yoghurt with chopped or puréed or stewed fruit like pear, mango or banana
Breast or bottle feed

Bedtime

Breast or bottle feed if required

Now You Can Give

- ❑ Wheat-based products like bread and pasta
- ❑ Dairy products like cheese and yoghurt
- ❑ Sieved berry fruits
- ❑ Citrus fruits
- ❑ Well-cooked egg
- ❑ Be careful with citrus fruits, dairy products, and cow's milk; these are very common causes of allergy.

Don't Give

- ❑ Soft ripened cheeses
- ❑ Chopped or whole nuts
- ❑ Salt
- ❑ Sugar
- ❑ Chilli or strong spices
- ❑ Tea

6

9 to 12 Months

Towards Family Meals

By around nine months, your baby will be well on the way to enjoying family meals. Life will be easier now as your baby is likely to be enjoying three meals a day and eating at times which are more in line with family mealtimes. Your baby should be able to cope with minced or finely chopped foods, thanks to her emerging teeth, which will help encourage chewing; she can swallow in a more coordinated way; and will start to get to grips with a cup, spoon and fork. By twelve months, your baby should be taking a good mixed diet from three meals and two to three healthy snacks daily.

Your baby's confidence will grow as she learns to pick up and grasp objects, too – as well as drop, bang and scrape them!

Food Fads and Fussy Eating

But, with this increasing confidence, you may find that she starts to exert her independence and refuse foods. If so, do try to be patient: just take whatever it is away and try offering it again another day, perhaps with one of your baby's favourite foods. You can't force a baby to eat and trying to do so will only lead to confrontation and frustration all round – it may even put your baby off trying new foods. The only way to avoid fussy eating habits is by encouragement and gentle persuasion. A healthy baby will not voluntarily starve herself and regular weighing at your child health clinic should help to reassure you that your baby is growing and developing normally. You can also take the opportunity to discuss any problems with your health visitor.

Tips to Prevent Fussy Feeding

- ❏ Make meals fun, offer a variety of foods and use colour, shapes, and different textures to add interest
- ❏ Set a good example: eat together if you can, and let your baby see you enjoying your food
- ❏ Allow plenty of time for meals
- ❏ Serve meals on colourful bowls and plates
- ❏ Encourage mealtimes with friends
- ❏ Serve meals at the table so your baby knows what to expect
- ❏ Don't offer a mountain of food – make portions small and offer seconds
- ❏ Encourage self-feeding where possible, but do be prepared for a mess

- Make sure your baby is sitting comfortably
- Offer your baby her favourite foods regularly
- Moisten foods with sauces and gravies (unsalted) to make sure they are not too dry and difficult to swallow

Your baby is an individual and, while some are big eaters, some will only eat small amounts, so do be guided by her appetite. Also, be aware that her appetite will change as she grows.

Not Yet

Your baby should be able to eat most foods now, but still avoid:

- salty, sugary and fatty foods
- hot spices like chilli
- whole nuts
- tea
- fizzy or adult drinks
- too many high-fibre foods
- soft ripened cheeses
- cow's milk products
- oranges and orange juice.

Dip It!

From around nine months, your baby will start to be able to use her thumb and forefinger to point to and pick up foods. Make use of this new skill by offering finger-foods that your baby can dip. Try mashing some ripe avocado with a sprinkling of lemon juice, or purée fruits and vegetables like carrot, pumpkin, sweet potato, apple, banana, and sieved raspberries. Try pouring natural yoghurt over grated, peeled cucumber or offer a cheese sauce.

Dunk-ables

Offer these snacks with interesting shapes to dip and dunk:

- long slices of banana and apple wheels
- cheese sticks, breadsticks and trimmed sticks of celery
- bread or toast soldiers
- toasted pitta triangles
- carrot batons
- pear, avocado, and cooked potato wedges
- trimmed green beans
- broccoli and cauliflower trees
- chunks of apricot and peach
- thin slices of melon
- cooked red, green, and white pasta shapes
- unsalted crackers
- cubed pieces of chicken.

Your baby should be having some drinks from a cup now. Try introducing a cup at lunchtime, then breakfast, and then with the evening bottle.

Weaning-at-a-glance Calendar:

Nine to Twelve Months

Your baby may not need a milk drink on waking, but do keep pace with your baby's individual needs.

Breakfast

Breakfast cereal or porridge with your baby's usual milk and fruit
Toast fingers
Breast or bottle feed

Lunch

Chopped meat, liver, chicken, fish, pulses or lentils or cheese with mashed vegetables and pasta, rice, potatoes or bread
Fingers of fruit with yoghurt or milk pudding
Water or fruit juice from a cup

Tea

Toast or bread with banana or yoghurt
Pasta with tomato sauce
Sandwiches
Potatoes with cheese sauce
Breast or bottle feed

Bedtime

Breast or bottle feed if required

Your baby may continue to sleep both morning and afternoon, or may start to grow out of one or more daytime sleeps. Continue to offer a drink of milk between breakfast and/or lunch if your baby wants it. Be careful with citrus fruits, dairy products, and cow's milk; these are very common causes of allergy. By 12 months, cows' milk can be used for purées or sauces.

Don't Give

- ☐ Whole or chopped nuts
- ☐ Salty, sugary or fatty foods
- ☐ Soft ripened cheeses
- ☐ Tea

Twelve Months: The Age of the Toddler

After a year, your baby can drink cow's milk as a main milk drink but will still need to drink around 350 ml (two thirds of a pint) per day. Many breastfed babies will continue with some breastfeeds well into the second year. You can continue to breastfeed as long as you and your baby want to. You probably won't need to prepare special meals now, as your baby can join in with family meals (remember that it would benefit every family member not to eat too much fat or sugar and enjoy more starchy foods, vegetables and fruits). Because your baby has high requirements for nutrient-packed foods, though, you should still offer a few (perhaps two or three) snacks like bread or fruit between meals.

II

Recipes

7

Guidelines Before You Begin

What You Need to Know Before You Start

Food Safety Tips

- ☐ To avoid the risk of food poisoning, wash all the equipment you use carefully in very hot water. Wash your baby's spoons, cups and bowls in hot water, and scald them with boiling water just before you use them. You don't need to sterilize this equipment.
- ☐ Don't keep half-eaten food. You can keep untouched portions in the fridge for up to 24 hours. Reheat the food thoroughly and cool it before giving it to your baby.
- ☐ Always wash your hands before touching foods and keep work surfaces clean and dry.
- ☐ If you are using food from the freezer, make sure it is completely thawed. Then boil it, stirring well to make sure it is heated right through. Let it cool before you give it to your baby.
- ☐ Never heat milk in a microwave.

- If you use a microwave, make sure the food is not too hot. Even if the cooking container is cool to the touch, the food may be hot in the middle.
- Check the 'use by' date on ready-made food before you give it to your baby.
- Never add solid food such as cereal to your baby's milk or drinks, because he could choke.
- Never leave your baby alone while he is eating.

What You Need to Make Your Own Baby Foods

Making your own baby foods is quick and easy and will start to condition your baby's tastes for more delicious family meals to come.

To make first foods, either peel, scrub or prepare your chosen fruit or vegetables. Cut into pieces, cover with a little water and steam, microwave or simmer gently. When cooked, add a little of the cooking water (which contains soluble vitamins) or your baby's usual milk.

Either push soft, cooked foods through a sieve using the back of a metal spoon, or blend larger quantities to a smooth, runny texture.

Preserve Those Vitamins

The way you prepare vegetables and fruits will affect their nutritional content. Water-soluble vitamins (such as vitamin C) are destroyed when vegetables are cut, boiled, or kept warm for long periods.

To maximize the nutritional content of foods:

- add the minimum of water (which should be boiling) to vegetables and fruits, cover and cook until just tender
- use the cooking water to make soups, sauces and gravies
- try steaming. It helps foods retain their delicate vitamins and it enhances natural flavours
- if you have a microwave, try using it to cook vegetables and fruits; just add a little water, cover with a lid in a suitable container, and cook until tender
- don't keep foods hot for long periods. If possible, serve soon after preparing
- offer some vegetables and fruits raw.

Frozen vegetables are often high in vitamins (sometimes more so than fresh produce that has been stored for long periods) because they are frozen soon after harvesting. Canned products are less nutritious.

First foods should be smooth, runny and bland. Later, when the teeth appear and biting and chewing become easier, foods can be mashed or grated.

8

First Food Recipes

Most of the recipes in this book use wholesome natural ingredients like vegetables and fruits, bread, rice and pulses, lean meat and fish. Only the minimum amount of sugar is added, and then only in the later stages of introducing your baby to a mixed diet. I have also made use, where possible, of more unusual or exotic produce to encourage your baby's love of a wide variety of foods. Many international dishes have been adapted so that they are suitable for babies and young children, while others have their origins closer to home.

You can make delicious family meals from most of these recipes by increasing the quantities (most are designed to make two to four portions, except the soups, which make up about 1½ to 2 pints). The fruit purées make great sauces for the rest of the family with yoghurt or fromage frais on breakfast cereals and porridge, or with custard or vanilla ice cream.

Initially, you can save time when cooking vegetables or fruits simply by removing cooked portions before the addition of salt or sugar and puréeing for your baby. Later on the recipes are designed to be suitable for babies and also to appeal to other family members, so you don't have to spend the whole day tied to the cooker.

Where Can You Start?

Manufactured baby rice (available from supermarkets and pharmacies) is a quick and convenient first food. To begin with you will only need very small amounts, so this is a good way to make up as little (or as much) as you need. Mix with cooled, boiled water, formula milk, or a little expressed breastmilk. Alternatively, you can make your own baby rice: just sieve or purée some cooked rice.

Making Your Own Babyfoods:

Saving Time

- ❏ Save time by making up purées in advance.
- ❏ When cooking vegetables for the family, take out a small portion and purée it for your baby.
- ❏ Remember not to add salt to your baby's portion.
- ❏ Freeze puréed portion in ice cube trays, or in yoghurt pots.
- ❏ When frozen, turn into a clean plastic bag and label.
- ❏ Defrost only as much as you need.

First Foods

These first purée recipes make around 5–6 fl oz of purée. Alternatively, vary the amount of vegetables and fruits and make up just enough for one portion if you wish. You can also save time by cooking the vegetables for the rest of the family, and just take out your baby's portion before seasoning. Cooking times are average and will vary slightly according to individual cooking equipment. If you use a microwave to prepare dishes, do allow the food to stand for a few minutes to complete cooking. You can store unused purée in the fridge for 24 hours or freeze for up to a month, unless the recipe states it is unsuitable for freezing.

Vegetable Purées

Carrot Purée

Wash and peel 100 g (4 oz) carrots and chop fine.

Place in a pan and cover with just a little boiling water. Cover and simmer for about 10 minutes or until tender. Purée with 2 to 3 table-spoons of the cooking water.

To microwave, place the carrots into a suitable dish. Add 2 to 3 tablespoons of cooled boiled water, cover with microwave film, pierce the film and cook for 3 to 4 minutes on full power. Allow to stand for a few minutes, then purée with a blender or push through a sieve, adding water to produce a smooth consistency.

Alternatively, for a creamy purée, drain the carrots after cooking and mix with three or four tablespoons of your baby's usual milk.

Swede

Wash and peel 100 g (4 oz) swedes and cut into chunks.

Place in a pan and cover with a little boiling water. Cover and cook for 10 minutes or so or until tender. Purée and add a little of your baby's usual milk for a smooth, runny consistency.

To microwave, place the swedes in a suitable container, cover with a little boiling water and microwave film. Pierce the film and cook on full power for 4 to 5 minutes. Mix with more boiled water or your baby's usual milk for a smooth consistency.

Parsnip

Wash and peel 100 g (4 oz) parsnips and chop into chunks.

Place in a pan with a little boiling water, cover and simmer for about 10 minutes or until cooked. Drain and purée, mixing with a little of your baby's usual milk until you have a smooth consistency.

To microwave, place in a microwavable bowl and add about 3 tablespoons of boiled cooled water. Cover with microwave film. Pierce the film and cook on full power for about 4 minutes. Drain, purée and mix with 2 to 3 tablespoons of your baby's usual milk.

Butternut Squash

A winter squash that resembles a large peanut, the sweet, mild flesh is also rich in beta carotene.

Cut a portion of butternut squash, peel and scoop out the seeds.

Place the pieces of squash in a pan, pour over a little boiling water and simmer gently for about 20 minutes or until tender. Drain and purée with a little of your baby's usual milk.

Alternatively, brush a portion of butternut squash with a little sunflower oil and place in an oven-proof dish. Bake in a moderate oven (Gas Mark 4/180°C/350°F) for about 50 minutes or until tender before you cut away the skin and purée.

Turnip

Wash and peel 100 g (4 oz) turnips and chop into chunks.

Place in a pan with just a little boiling water, cover and simmer for about 10 minutes or until cooked. Drain and purée, mixing with a little of your baby's usual milk until you have a smooth consistency.

To microwave, place in a microwavable bowl and add about 3 tablespoons of boiled cooled water. Cover with microwave film. Pierce the film and cook on full power for about 4 minutes. Drain and purée, adding a little of the cooking water if necessary.

Sweet Potato

The sweet potato has a lovely sweet taste and is also bursting with vitamins and pigments like beta carotene.

Peeling after cooking will help to retain its delicate colour. To prepare, wash 100 g (4 oz) sweet potato and slit the skin. Bake in the skin in a moderate oven (Gas Mark 4/180°C/350°F) for about 40 minutes or until tender. Cool slightly and peel then purée.

To microwave, cut into large chunks and place in a suitable dish. Cover with microwave film, pierce the film and microwave on high for about 10 minutes or until tender. Allow to stand, peel off the skin and purée with a little of your baby's usual milk.

Potato

Wash 100 g (4 oz) potatoes and cut into chunks.

Place in a pan, adding a little boiling water to just cover the pota-to. Cover and simmer gently for about 10 minutes or until tender. Allow to cool and peel off the skin.

To bake, place the unpeeled, washed sweet potato in a suitable oven-proof dish and bake in a moderate oven (Gas Mark 5/190°C/375°F) for about 30 minutes or until tender. Allow to cool slightly before peeling off the skin. Then purée or pass through a sieve and add a little of your baby's usual milk until you have a smooth consistency.

Green Beans

Choose young beans which have a sweeter taste and are more tender.

Trim the beans and cut away any stringy parts, cut into 2.5-cm (1-inch) pieces. Place in a pan and half-cover with cold water. Bring to the boil, cover and simmer for about 10 minutes. Cool and purée, adding some of the cooking water if necessary for a smooth texture.

Courgette

A member of the summer squash family, courgettes have soft skins so they don't have to be peeled before cooking. The seeds are edible.

Wash, trim and slice 100 g (4 oz) courgettes. Place in a pan with a little boiling water. Cover and simmer gently for about 8 to 10 min-utes. Drain and purée, adding some of the cooking water if necessary.

To microwave, place the pieces of courgette in a microwavable dish, cover with microwave film. Pierce the film and microwave on high for about 4 minutes or until tender. Allow to cool, then purée.

Green Pea Purée

Frozen peas are always a nutritious standby for all the family, even the youngest members!

Place the required amount of peas in a pan and cover with a little boiling water. Bring to the boil, reduce the heat and simmer for 2 or 3 minutes. Cool and purée, adding a little of the cooking water if necessary.

Spring Green Purée

Choose firm young leaves for a sweeter flavour.

Wash the required amount of spring greens and remove the tough stalks. Shred and place in a pan. Add a little boiling water, cover and simmer for about 8 minutes or until tender. Drain and purée, adding a little of the cooking water if necessary.

Broccoli

A good source of beta carotene and vitamin C. Cook for the minimum amount of time to retain the maximum amounts of nutrients.

Place the required amount of small broccoli florets in a microwavable container, add a little boiling water and cover with microwave film. Pierce the film and microwave on high for about 3 to 4 minutes or until tender. Drain, reserving the cooking liquid, and purée, adding some cooking water if necessary to produce a smooth, runny consistency.

Alternatively, steam the florets for about 10 to 15 minutes before you purée.

Cauliflower

Choose the freshest cauliflower and try steaming or microwaving cauliflower florets to help retain the vitamins.

Wash and cut into small florets. Place the required amount of cauliflower florets in a microwavable container. Add a small amount of boiling water and cover with microwave film. Pierce the film and microwave on high for about 3 to 4 minutes or until tender. Drain, reserving the cooking liquid, and purée, adding some cooking water if necessary to produce a smooth, runny consistency.

Alternatively, steam the florets for about 10 to 15 minutes before you purée.

Fruit Purées

Eating Apple

Choose a sweet dessert apple for this purée.

Wash, peel and core a ripe apple. Cut into dice. Place in a pan with 2 to 3 tablespoons of water and bring to the boil. Cover and simmer until soft. Cool and drain, then purée with a hand blender or push through a sieve using the back of a metal spoon, adding a little of the cooking water if necessary.

To microwave, peel, core and chop the apple. Place the fruit in a suitable dish, add 2 to 3 tablespoons of water and cover with microwave film. Pierce the film and cook on full power for about 2 minutes or until tender. Allow to cool, then purée.

Pear

Wash, peel and cut a ripe fruit into quarters. Core the fruit and cut into chunks. Add 2 tablespoons of boiling water, cover and simmer for about 10 minutes or until tender. Cool, then sieve or purée to a smooth, runny consistency, adding some of the cooking water if necessary.

To microwave, place the pieces of pear into a microwavable dish. Cover with microwave film. Pierce and microwave on high for about 4 minutes. Leave to cool, then purée.

TIP
Make up extra puréed fruits for older babies, children and the rest of the family to enjoy with yoghurt or as a topping for breakfast cereals or with ice cream.

Banana

Cut a small piece of ripe banana (the fruit is ripe when the skin is freckled) and mash well to form a runny, smooth texture. Serve soon after preparation, as banana soon discolours. Banana does not freeze well.

9

5 to 6 Months

Now, as your baby begins to get used to a mixed diet in addition to milk, you can start to increase the variety of foods offered and mix foods rather than offering single purées.

Vegetable Dishes

Pumpkin and Spinach Purée

    100 g (4 oz) pumpkin flesh, cut into dice
    sunflower oil
    100 g (4 oz) spinach leaves
    milk as needed

Brush the pumpkin with a little sunflower oil, place in an oven-proof dish, cover with foil and bake in the oven (Gas Mark 4/180°C/350°F) for 40–50 minutes or until tender. Cool and purée.

To prepare the spinach, remove the stalks and place in a pan. Add just a little boiling water, cover and simmer for about 5 minutes. Drain well. Purée and mix with the pumpkin, adding a little of your baby's usual milk if necessary.

Tomato, Green Bean and Baby Rice Dinner

75 g (3 oz) green beans, washed, trimmed and chopped
boiling water
1 tomato, peeled, de-seeded and chopped
a little prepared baby rice

Place the beans in a pan and add a little boiling water. Bring to the boil, cover and simmer for about 5 minutes. Add the tomato and cook for another 5 minutes or so. Drain and purée, reserving some of the cooking water. Stir in a little prepared baby rice and some cooking water if necessary until you have the desired consistency.

Creamy Carrots and Parsnips with Nutmeg

100 g (4 oz) carrots
50 g (2 oz) parsnips
boiling water
a little sunflower margarine or butter
pinch of nutmeg
milk

Wash, peel and chop the carrots and parsnips and place in a pan.

Add a little boiling water, cover and simmer for about 10 minutes or until tender. Drain, add the margarine or butter and purée with the nutmeg and a little of your baby's usual milk until you have the desired consistency.

To microwave, place the vegetables in a microwave dish, add a little boiling water, cover with microwave film and microwave on high for about 8 to 10 minutes or until tender. Purée with the nutmeg, adding a little of your baby's usual milk.

Mixed Root Vegetable Purée

Mix and match whatever root vegetables your baby (and your family) enjoy. Try adding one or more orange vegetables, like sweet potato or carrot, for a brightly coloured purée. A meal in itself for a young baby, but for older children and adults, serve with meat, chicken or lentil casserole and a green vegetable.

Prepare your selection of mixed root vegetables, such as pumpkin, potato, swede, parsnips, carrot, sweet potato. Peel, wash and chop the vegetables and place them in a pan with a little boiling water. Cover and cook until tender. Drain, reserving some of the cooking liquid. Mash or purée until smooth, adding a little of your baby's usual milk and a little of the cooking water if necessary to produce a smooth consistency.

Spinach Purée with Nutmeg

100 g (4 oz) young spinach leaves, stalks removed
1 tsp margarine or butter
pinch grated nutmeg
milk as needed

Steam, microwave or boil the spinach until tender. Drain carefully and squeeze out excess moisture. Add the margarine or butter and the nutmeg and purée, adding a little of your baby's usual milk to obtain the required consistency.

Sweet Pepper

Peppers are packed with vitamin C, but red or orange varieties are sweeter than green peppers and so they may be more appealing to your baby at first. But, even though they are sweet, peppers can have a very strong, distinctive taste, so you may want to mix some pepper purée with something a little more bland, like potato.

To prepare, peel the skin off using a sharp potato peeler. Trim, slice in half and remove the seeds and pith. Cut into strips and steam, boil or microwave until tender. Purée.

Roasted Pumpkin with Cinnamon

Another much under-used vegetable, cooked pumpkin has a delicious sweet flavour and, when puréed or in soups, has a wonderful velvety texture. For older members of the family, serve with roasted meat or a poultry or bean casserole.

1 tsp sunflower margarine or butter
$\frac{1}{2}$ tsp cinnamon powder
175 g (6 oz) piece of pumpkin
milk

Melt the margarine or butter in a pan or in a bowl in a microwave. Sprinkle the cinnamon powder over the melted margarine or butter.

Place the pumpkin in a large piece of foil (enough to completely cover the pumpkin). Pour the melted margarine or butter over the pumpkin and bake in a moderate oven (Gas Mark 5/190°C/375°F) for 40–50 minutes or until cooked through. Cool and scoop out the flesh and purée. Add a little of your baby's usual milk if the mixture is dry.

Vegetable Combinations

Sweet Potato and Carrot

Try this bright orange purée packed with vitamins and minerals by mixing together purées of sweet potato and carrot. Sweet potato will retain its attractive colour if you bake it in its jacket. When cooked, scoop out the orange flesh, mash well with a little of your baby's usual milk and mix with puréed carrot in equal quantities.

Sweet Potato and Potato

Make a sweet version of traditional mashed potato by mixing equal quantities of mashed potato with sweet potato. You can vary the sweetness of the mash by adding more sweet potato if you wish.

Creamed Parsnips with Spinach

Use equal quantities of parsnips and spinach or, if the taste of spinach is too strong for your baby, use more parsnips.

Cook and purée parsnips in the usual way. Then, prepare the spinach. Choose a few fresh young spinach leaves, cut out any tough stalks and steam, microwave or boil in a covered pan until tender. Drain well in a colander or on kitchen paper, squeezing out the excess water. Purée.

Combine the puréed spinach with the cooked parsnips, adding a little of your baby's usual milk.

Potato and Watercress Purée

1 small potato, peeled, scrubbed and diced
butter or margarine
milk
1 small handful watercress, washed
cooking water as needed

Cook the potato in the usual way, then purée with a little butter or margarine and your baby's usual milk.

Pick off the leaves from the watercress and discard the stems. Steam in a little boiling water for 4 or 5 minutes. Drain and purée the watercress and stir into the potato mixture, adding a little of the cooking water if necessary.

Clapshot (Potato and Swede Purée)

This Scottish purée of potato and swede is traditionally served with oat cakes or with meat and poultry with a sprinkling of browned onions.

50 g (2 oz) swede, peeled and chopped
50 g (2 oz) potatoes, peeled and chopped
boiling water
dab of butter or sunflower margarine
milk

Cook the swede and potatoes in a little boiling water in a covered pan for about 10 minutes or until tender. Drain and purée with a dab of butter or margarine and a little of your baby's usual milk if desired.

Potato with Celeriac

With its unusual appearance, celeriac is a much under-used vegetable in this country, but its sweet distinctive taste should make it a hit with all the family.

50 g (2 oz) potato, peeled and diced
50 g (2 oz) celeriac, cut into slices, peeled and diced

Boil potato and celeriac in water for about 15–20 minutes or until tender. Purée and serve
For older members of the family, stir in a little crushed garlic.

Mix and Match

Be bold and mix vegetables and fruits together, even those that you would not normally feel go together, such as carrot and apple, courgette and banana, pears and peas, sweet potato and parsnip.

Fruit Dishes

Special Cherry and Banana Rice

six ripe cherries
2 tbsp boiling water
half a ripe banana, mashed
a little baby rice to mix
sugar if needed

Choose a ripe banana and ripe cherries for a sweeter taste. You may need to add a sprinkling of sugar if the fruit is too tart.

Wash the cherries in a sieve under running water. Place the cherries in a pan and add the boiling water. Cover and simmer for about 5 minutes. Remove the cherry pips and cool slightly. Pass the cherries through a sieve to remove the skins. Mix with the banana purée and stir in a little baby rice. Sweeten with a little sugar if the mixture is too sharp. For older members of the family, you can replace baby rice with rice pudding.

Melon

There are many types of melon available in the shops and supermarkets today, but you may want to try cantaloupe melon first – it has a lovely sweet taste and is also bursting with beta carotene.

Wash and cut a melon into two. Scoop out the seeds and discard. Cut a suitable sized wedge and peel away the skin before cutting into chunks. Sieve or purée until you have a smooth, runny texture. Melon does not freeze well.

Mango

Sweet, fragrant mango contains beta carotene and vitamin C. Its distinctive flavour is sure to become a favourite!

To prepare, wash a ripe, unblemished mango. Then, using a sharp knife, cut lengthwise along each side as near as possible to the stone. Cut the mango into criss-cross sections and scoop out the flesh. Peel away the remaining skin and purée the required amount of mango flesh.

Paw Paw (Papaya)

A sweet, delicious treat for all the family!

To prepare, choose a ripe, unblemished fruit (press gently at each end, a papaya is ripe when it gives slightly) and cut lengthways. Scoop out the dark seeds and, using a sharp knife, cut away the skin. Then, purée the amount required for your baby until smooth.

Melon/Mango/Paw Paw (Papaya)

Simply peel and scoop out and/or discard the pips or stone. Steam or microwave for 2 or 3 minutes and sieve or purée to form a smooth, runny texture.

When your baby is about six months old, you will not have to cook these delicious fruits, simply prepare (purée, mash, chop or cut into slices) and serve alone or with a thick yoghurt or custard.

Apricot/Peach/Nectarine/Plum

Slit the skins and then plunge into boiling water for 2 or 3 minutes. Allow to cool slightly before peeling off the skin (you may need to re-immerse the fruit for a little longer if the skin is still not loose).

Steam or microwave with a little cooled, boiled water until tender; then purée.

Dried Fruit Purée

Wash a mixture of apricots, peaches and prunes (or use a single type of fruit) and leave to soak in water overnight.

Discard the water and cook in a little boiling water until succulent. Cool and sieve (to remove the skins, which can be a little tough and difficult for a small baby to digest).

You can mix this dried fruit purée with puréed fresh fruit or, later on, with Greek yoghurt, fromage frais or unsweetened custard. Alternatively, add a little to your baby's breakfast cereal.

Note: dried fruits, especially prunes, have a laxative effect, so use sparingly, especially for small babies.

Avocado

Your baby may enjoy the mild taste and velvety texture of avocado. Later, she will enjoy holding slices of avocado as finger-food.

Choose a ripe avocado, peel and remove the stone. Mash or purée a portion to obtain a smooth purée. Avocados are very rich, so you may want to mix avocado with another vegetable or fruit purée.

Avocado and Pear Mix

Avocado has a delicious, mild taste, but it does contain a lot of oil, so your baby may find it a little rich on its own.

For a satisfying fruity purée, peel, core and wash a ripe eating pear, then steam, microwave or boil it until tender. Purée.

Mix the puréed pear with a little mashed avocado pear.

Banana Rice with Cinnamon

Make up some baby rice according to the instructions on the packet using some of your baby's usual milk. Add to this a little mashed banana and a pinch of powdered cinnamon.

10

6 to 9 Months

Your baby will now be able to progress to slightly coarser purées. Remember, though, that your baby is an individual, so do be guided by your baby's individual needs.

Basic Stocks and Sauces

Now your baby can enjoy more family meals, these basic stocks and sauces will be useful when making meals for all the family which your baby will also enjoy.

White Chicken Stock

A good stock adds body and flavour to your cooking, and is the basis of a good soup, casserole or stew. And, by making your own stock, you can be sure that it is free of salt and other additives which may be present in stock cubes.

1 kg (2 lb) raw chicken bones
2 litres (4 pints) of water
250 g (½ lb) of carrot, onion, celery, leek, swede and turnip
fresh herbs such as parsley and thyme
1 bay leaf
3 or 4 peppercorns

Clean the chicken bones and remove any fat or skin before placing in a large pan. Add the water and simmer gently for 30 minutes, then skim off any fat.

Chop the mixed vegetables and add to the pan together with the herbs and peppercorns. Simmer gently for 2 hours.

Cool and strain, discarding the bones and vegetables. Skim off any visible fat.

You can keep this stock in the fridge for 2 days or, when cool, pour into airtight containers and freeze.

To make a darker stock with a stronger flavour, brown the bones by frying in a little sunflower oil first.

Vegetable Stock

Use this vegetable stock when making meat-free dishes, sauces, gravies and soups, or use with meat-based dishes if you wish. Freeze the stock and use when needed.

500 g (1 lb) mixed vegetables (onion, carrot, turnip, swede, celery, leek)
sunflower oil for frying
2 litres (4 pints) water
fresh parsley and thyme or other herbs such as oregano
1 bay leaf
3 or 4 black peppercorns

Sauté the chopped, cleaned vegetables in the oil in a covered pan for a few minutes without browning.

Add the water, herbs and peppercorns, cover and simmer gently for about 2 hours.

Cool, strain and discard the vegetables and herbs. Refrigerate.

Skim off any fat before using.

Tomato Sauce

A delicious, versatile sauce, the tangy taste blends well with almost everything – try it with cooked pulses such as red kidney beans or haricot beans, with chicken, meat, fish, pasta, rice or couscous!

25 g (1 oz) margarine or butter
1 400 g (16–oz) tin of tomatoes
50 g (2 oz) chopped carrots
50 g (2 oz) chopped onion
25 g (1 oz) celery trimmed and chopped
1 clove garlic, crushed
25 g (1 oz) flour
250 ml (9 fl oz) heated, unsalted vegetable or chicken stock
1 tsp tomato purée

Cook the tinned tomatoes, carrots, onion and celery in the butter or margarine in a heavy-bottomed pan for a few minutes, then add the garlic (adding it after the vegetables are cooked will help to prevent it burning).

Add the flour and mix well. Pour in the hot stock, stirring constantly. Then, add the tomato purée and simmer gently in a covered pan for 30 minutes.

Cool and pass through a sieve or blender to a smooth consistency.

White Sauce

This basic white sauce recipe is thickened with a *roux* (a mixture of equal quantities of flour and margarine or butter). You can use it as a base for other sauces and even for some soups.

> 50 g (2 oz) sunflower margarine or butter
> 50 g (2 oz) flour
> 600 ml (1 pint) warm milk

Melt the margarine or butter slowly to prevent burning in a heavy-bottomed pan. Add the flour and mix together with a whisk and cook gently for a minute or two. Gradually add the warmed milk, whisking all the time to prevent any lumps. Simmer gently without boiling for a few minutes or so.

For a thinner sauce, halve the quantities of flour and margarine or butter but keep the amount of milk the same.

Soups and Stews

Butternut Squash and Orange Soup

> sunflower or olive oil for frying
> 1 medium onion, chopped fine
> 1 medium butternut squash, peeled, deseeded and chopped
> 850 ml (1½ pints) vegetable stock
> 1 tbsp fresh coriander
> juice of one orange
> ½ tsp orange rind
> Greek yoghurt, plain fromage frais or single cream

Fry the onion without browning (about five minutes). Add the chopped squash and cook for another minute or two. Pour on the stock and simmer for 15–20 minutes or until the squash is tender.

Cool slightly, add the coriander, juice and rind and whizz in a blender until smooth. Return the soup to a pan and heat through.

Serve with Greek yoghurt, fromage frais or cream.

Irish Stew

A simple to make but delicious traditional dish.

    350 g (12 oz) diced lamb
    1 tbsp fresh parsley
    1 onion cut into rings
    350 g (12 oz) potatoes, washed and cut into slices
    150 ml (5 fl oz) water

Place a layer of the diced meat in an oven-proof dish, sprinkle over a little chopped parsley, top with a layer of onions and then the slices of potato. Continue layering the ingredients in this way, finishing with a layer of potato. Pour on the water.

Cover and cook (on Gas Mark 3/160°C/325°F) for 1½ hours or until the meat is tender. Purée or mash as required for your baby.

Minestrone

A hearty and classic Italian dish that babies and the rest of the family will love. For older members of the family, add grated Parmesan or Pecorino cheese and serve with fresh bread to dip and dunk.

50 g (2 oz) onion, chopped

sunflower oil for frying

1 clove of garlic, crushed

850 ml (1¹/₂ pints) chicken or vegetable stock

50 g (2 oz) carrot, chopped

50 g (2 oz) potatoes, peeled and chopped

50 g (2 oz) white part of leek, chopped

1 × 5 oz tin tomatoes, blended with their juice

1 tsp tomato purée

50 g (2 oz) spaghetti, broken into small pieces

25 g (1 oz) frozen green beans, chopped

2 tsp chopped parsley

Sauté the onion in a covered pan over a gentle heat in a little oil, without browning. Add the garlic and the stock and simmer gently for about 20 minutes.

Add the carrots, potato, leeks and blended tomatoes, tomato purée and spaghetti broken into small pieces and continue to simmer gently for a further 10 minutes.

Add the beans and cook for a further few minutes. Finally, sprinkle over the chopped parsley and serve.

Carrot Soup with Spinach and Lentils

This soup is thickened with lentils and has a lovely sweet taste.

1 small onion, chopped

sunflower oil

200 g (8 oz) carrots, peeled and sliced

100 g (4 oz) red lentils picked over for any small stones

850 ml (1¹/₂ pints) vegetable or chicken stock

100 g (4 oz) mixed root vegetables (such as swede, turnip, parsnip)

100 g (4 oz) young spinach leaves
2 tbsp fresh parsley, chopped

Sauté the onion in a little sunflower oil without browning. Add the carrots and cook gently for another 5 minutes.

Wash the lentils in a sieve under running water and add to the carrots and onion. Pour on the stock, bring to the boil and simmer gently for about 25 minutes.

Wash the spinach leaves and remove any tough stalks. Add to the soup with the chopped parsley. Take off the burner. Cool and whizz in a blender until smooth.

Serve with a swirl of fromage frais and fresh bread.

Tomato Soup with Basil

2 shallots or small onions, chopped
olive oil for frying
500 g (20 oz) tomatoes, peeled and chopped
1 tbsp tomato purée
850 ml (1½ pints) vegetable or chicken stock
2 shallots, chopped
2 tbsp fresh basil, chopped

Sauté the shallots in the olive oil in a large pan for 5 minutes without browning.

Stir in the tomatoes and the tomato purée and cook for another 4 minutes.

Pour on the stock, cover and simmer for 30 minutes. Sprinkle over the chopped basil.

Cool slightly and purée before serving with fresh bread to dunk.

Leek and Potato Soup

A hearty soup that is a firm family favourite in our household!

    1 small onion, chopped
    2 leeks (white part), trimmed, cleaned and chopped
    sunflower oil for frying
    3 medium-sized potatoes, peeled and chopped
    850 ml (1½ pints) chicken or vegetable stock
    2 tsp Greek yoghurt or cream
    chopped parsley and chives

Sauté the onion and the leeks in the sunflower oil without browning for 5 minutes or so.

Add the potatoes and the stock and simmer gently for 30 minutes or so. Cool slightly and purée.

Just before serving, stir in the Greek yoghurt or cream and sprinkle with the chopped herbs.

For a thicker purée, add less stock.

Creamy Pea Soup

    1 small onion, chopped
    sunflower oil for frying
    500 g (20 oz) frozen peas
    parsley and thyme
    850 ml (1½ pints) vegetable or chicken stock
    3 × 15 ml (3 tbsp) Greek yoghurt or single cream
    fresh mint, chopped

Sauté the onion in a little sunflower oil without browning for 5 minutes until soft.

Add the peas, herbs and stock and simmer gently for 30 minutes.

Cool slightly, remove the herbs and purée. Stir in the yoghurt or cream and add a little mint.

Carrot and Parsnip Soup

Sweet and hearty.

1 tbsp olive oil
1 onion, chopped fine
1 clove garlic, crushed
500 g (1 lb) carrots, sliced
350 g (12oz) parsnips, sliced
1.2 litres (2 pints) vegetable stock
1 bay leaf
2 tbsp fresh parsley, chopped

Heat the oil in a large pan and add the onion and garlic. Fry for 5 minutes to soften without colouring.

Add the carrots and parsnips and cook for a further 5 minutes.

Add the stock and simmer for 20 minutes until the vegetables are tender.

When cool, transfer to a blender and purée. Return to the pan and season.

Add the chopped parsley just before serving.

Chicken Meals

Chicken Liver and Apple Casserole

Chicken liver is very economical and its milk taste makes it a good introduction to liver for your baby. The addition of apple will add a little sweetness which babies enjoy.

sunflower oil for frying
50 g (2 oz) chicken liver
1 medium potato, peeled and chopped
1 small carrot, peeled and chopped
100 ml (4 fl oz) unsalted chicken or vegetable stock
half an eating apple, puréed
chopped parsley

Clean the chicken livers, removing any fat or gristle before slicing. Sauté the liver in a little oil, then add the potato and carrot and cook for minute or two more.

Add the stock and simmer for 10 minutes. Stir in the apple purée and heat through. Add a little chopped parsley.

To serve, purée, mash or chop as necessary. Serve with pasta shapes, rice or fresh bread.

Chicken with Peaches and Pasta

1 chicken breast (free-range if possible)
flour for coating
sunflower oil for frying
1 small onion, chopped

100 ml (4 fl oz) chicken or vegetable stock
half a ripe peach
boiling water
50 g (2 oz) small pasta shapes, cooked

Cut the chicken into strips and coat with flour (place the flour in a clean polythene bag, add the chicken strips and shake gently to coat). Dust off the excess flour. Fry the onion and chicken in a little sunflower oil for 3 or 4 minutes over a medium heat.

Add the stock and simmer gently for 20 minutes.

Slit the skin on the peach and place in a little boiling water for a minute or two. Then, peel off the skin and chop into small pieces. Add the peach to the chicken mixture and cook for a minute or two.

Add the cooked pasta, stir and warm through. Serve.

Meat Meals

Meaty Tomato, Courgette and Pasta

100 g (4 oz) lean beef, cubed
sunflower oil for frying
50 g (2 oz) courgettes, chopped
200 ml (7 fl oz) vegetable stock
50 g (2 oz) fresh tomato, peeled, de-seeded and chopped
50 g (2 oz) pasta shapes, cooked
parsley

Sauté the beef in a little oil until just browned, add the chopped courgette and continue cooking for a minute or two.

Pour in the stock and the tomato and simmer gently for another 10 minutes or so. Stir in the cooked pasta shapes and add some chopped parsley. Purée or chop and serve with green beans or peas.

VARIATION

You can use cubed lamb for this dish if you prefer.

Shepherds Pie with Parsnip and Potato Mash

Your baby may enjoy the sweet taste of the mash (from the parsnip) teamed with mince in gravy. If you wish, you can use minced lamb or minced Quorn instead. You can also add more vegetables to the meat to boost your baby's (and your family's) intake.

sunflower oil for frying
1 small onion, peeled and chopped
1 carrot, peeled and diced
200 g (8 oz) lean minced beef/lamb or Quorn
2 tsp plain flour
150 ml (5 fl oz) chicken stock
200 g (8 oz) potatoes, peeled and diced
200 g (8 oz) parsnips, peeled and diced
pat of butter
1 tbsp milk

Fry the onion and carrot in a little sunflower oil over a medium heat until the onion is translucent (about 5 minutes).

Add the meat and sprinkle over the flour, stirring well. Pour in the stock, cover and simmer for half an hour.

Cook the potatoes and parsnips in a little boiling water or in the microwave. When tender, drain and mash with a little butter (or sunflower oil or margarine) and a tablespoon of milk until smooth.

Pile the mash over the meat mixture and cook in a moderate oven (Gas Mark 4/180°C/350°F) for 20 minutes.

Serve with a mixture of vegetables.

Navarin of Lamb

This is a classic French lamb and vegetable stew. It's easy to make and it is delicious!

sunflower oil for frying
1 small onion
500 g (1 lb) lean lamb, cubed
600 ml (1 pint) vegetable stock
2 tsp tomato purée
150 ml (5 fl oz) pure unsweetened apple juice
100 g (4 oz) each carrots, peas, turnip and swede, cut into chunks
1 tbsp flour

Fry the onion in a large pan; add the meat and brown.

Add the stock, tomato purée and apple juice, bring to the boil, cover and simmer very gently for 1 hour or until the meat is tender.

Cook the vegetables in a little boiling water (or steam or microwave) until just tender. Drain and reserve.

Take a little of the gravy from the stock mixture; mix with the flour in a cup until smooth. Pour the flour mixture slowly back into the pan, stirring all the time to prevent any lumps forming. Cook for another 5 minutes.

A few minutes before you are ready to serve, add the vegetables to the stock mixture. Adjust the consistency to your baby's needs.

Serve with mashed or baked potatoes and butternut squash or baked pumpkin.

Fish Meals

Cooking Fresh or Frozen Fish

Fish is cooked when the colour changes from translucent to opaque and the fish will flake easily. Cooking times will vary according to the amount and thickness of the fish.

Steaming

Steaming fish helps it retain moisture and preserve delicate flavours. Place in a bamboo steamer and place over a pan with about 5 cm (2 inches) of hot water. Alternatively, pour the water into a pan and place the fish in a metal sieve and cover with a tight-fitting lid.

Microwaving

A quick way to cook fish, this method also retains delicate flavours. Simply place on a microwave-proof dish, cover and cook.

Baking

Place in a greased ovenproof dish (using sunflower oil or butter), cover with buttered foil and bake gently (Gas Mark 4/180°C/350°F). Do take care not to overcook, as the fish will dry out.

Fruity White Fish with Cheese

100 g (4 oz) white fish fillet (such as haddock, cod or coley)
dot of sunflower margarine or butter
1 tbsp pure unsweetened apple juice
100 ml (4 fl oz) white sauce
25 g (1 oz) grated Cheddar cheese

Dot the fish with a little margarine or butter and pour on the apple juice. Cook by steaming or within two plates in the microwave for 2 or 3 minutes, or wrapped in foil in a medium oven (Gas Mark 4/180°C/350°F) for 20 minutes.

Make up the white sauce (see page 88); stir in the grated cheese. Drain the liquid from the cooked fish and pour slowly into the cheese sauce, whisking all the time. Carefully flake the fish to remove any bones; pour the sauce over it.

Serve with mashed potatoes and green beans or peas.

Baked Haddock with Fennel and Chives

100 g (4 oz) haddock
a dot of butter oil or margarine
a squeeze of lemon juice
a quarter of a bulb of fennel
boiling water
100 ml (4 fl oz) white sauce
1 tsp chives, snipped

Wrap the fish in greased foil, dot with margarine or butter and squeeze over a little fresh lemon juice. Wrap the foil over the fish and bake in a moderate oven (Gas Mark 4/180°C/350°F) for about 10 minutes or until the fish flakes easily.

Cut the fennel into pieces and cook in a little boiling water in a covered pan for about 10 minutes or until tender. Drain, cool and purée.

Warm the white sauce and add to it the snipped chives and stir into the fennel purée. Pour the sauce over the fish and serve with vegetables and potato. Adjust the consistency to suit your baby.

Plaice with Parsley and Chive Sauce

100 g (4 oz) fillet of plaice
dot of margarine or butter
100 ml (4 fl oz) white sauce
2 tsp chopped fresh parsley
1 tsp chopped chives

Dot the fish with a little margarine or butter and cook by placing between two plates over a pan of simmering water for 4 or 5 minutes, or in a microwave for 2 or 3 minutes. Flake the fish carefully and set aside.

Make the white sauce up as usual (see page 88) and stir in the chopped herbs.

Add the fish to the sauce and mash or purée.

Fish with Orange Sauce

50 g (2 oz) white fish such as haddock or whiting
1 tbsp freshly squeezed orange juice
100 ml (4 fl oz) white sauce
fresh parsley, chopped

Steam the fish or cook in a microwave until just done, then flake and remove any bones. Place in a saucepan.

Whisk the orange juice with the white sauce (see page 88) and pour over the fish. Simmer very gently for about 5 minutes.

Sprinkle on the chopped parsley just before serving.

Serve with rice, pasta or mashed potatoes and vegetables.

Haddock Fish Cakes with Parsley and Spring Onions

The mild taste of these fish cakes makes it appealing to young babies and the green colour comes from plenty of chopped parsley.

100 g (4 oz) potatoes
butter or margarine and milk
100 g (4 oz) cooked white fish, flaked and bones removed
1 tbsp chopped parsley
1 tsp fresh lemon juice
flour as needed
beaten egg for binding
toasted breadcrumbs for coating
sunflower oil for frying

Wash, peel and cook the potatoes in a little fast boiling water in a covered pan for 15 minutes, until tender.

Mash with a little butter or margarine and milk and add the fish, parsley and lemon juice. Mix well.

With floured hands, divide the mixture into eight small cakes, shaped and flattened into rounds. Brush each cake on each side with a little beaten egg, then dip into the breadcrumbs.

Fry in a little sunflower oil for about 4 minutes, turning once. When cooked, remove the fish cakes and drain on kitchen paper.

Serve with carrots and broccoli trees and some fresh tomato sauce.

Tuna Broccoli Bake

1 large tin tuna, drained and flaked
200 ml (7 fl oz) white sauce
50 g (2 oz) Gruyere cheese, grated
150 g (6 oz) broccoli florets, cooked
100 g (4 oz) cooked, diced potatoes

Combine the tuna, white sauce, grated cheese and broccoli in a large ovenproof dish. Sprinkle on the potatoes and cook in a medium hot oven (Gas Mark 5/190°C/375°F) for 25 minutes until golden. Mash to the required consistency and serve with peas or other vegetables.

Vegetable Meals

Cauliflower Cheese

100 g (4 oz) cauliflower, cooked
100 ml (4 fl oz) white sauce
25 g (1 oz) grated Cheddar cheese

Make up the white sauce as on page 88, adding the cheese at the last minute and stirring in until smooth.

Pour the cheese sauce over the cooked cauliflower. Purée, mash or chop as desired.

Baked Beans and Cheesy Toast

2 tbsp baked beans with sauce
1 slice wholemeal toast
grated Cheddar cheese

Mash the beans. Toast the bread and pile the beans on top. Sprinkle with the cheese and warm under the grill until bubbling. Cut into fingers and serve warm.

Cheesy Lentils with Carrot

50 g (2 oz) red lentils
100 g (4 oz) carrots, peeled and chopped
100 ml (4 fl oz) water
1 tbsp grated Cheddar cheese
milk as needed

Pick over the lentils to remove any stones and rinse thoroughly in cold running water. Place in a pan of boiling water. Bring to the boil, cover and simmer for 30 minutes, adding more water if required.

Add the carrots and simmer for a further 10 minutes or so until both the lentils and carrots are tender. Drain.

Stir in some grated cheese while the carrot/lentil mixture is still warm. Purée or mash to the required consistency, adding some of your baby's usual milk if required.

Baked Potatoes with Cheesy Chives

1 medium potato
butter or sunflower margarine
1 tbsp Greek yoghurt
1 tbsp grated Cheddar cheese
1 tsp snipped chives

Wash the potato and dry with kitchen paper. Prick the potato all over with a fork. Place on a baking tray and bake in a moderate oven for about 30 minutes.

Meanwhile, mix together the yoghurt, cheese and chives.

Remove the potato from the oven. Cut in half and scoop out the flesh. Place the butter or margarine in the potato skin. Mix the potato flesh with the yoghurt and cheese mixture and pile it back into the potato. Cook for a further 10 minutes or until warmed through.

Mash to the required consistency, discarding the potato skin if you wish.

Pasta with Creamy Leeks and Tomato

    25 g (1 oz) tagliatelle pasta
    50 g (2 oz) white part of leek, washed and chopped
    margarine or butter for frying
    1 tomato, peeled, de-seeded and chopped
    50 ml (2 fl oz) white sauce

Cook the pasta in plenty of fast boiling water until tender (about 8–10 minutes). Drain and reserve.

Sauté the leek in a little margarine or butter for 2 minutes or until translucent, then add the tomato and cook for a further 2 minutes. Take off the heat and stir in the white sauce.

Purée (for young babies) or chop or serve as is for older children and adults.

Serve with green beans or peas.

Pasta with Tomato Sauce

    25 g (1 oz) pasta shapes
    100 ml (4 fl oz) tomato sauce (see recipe on page 87)
    chopped parsley, to serve

Cook the pasta in plenty of boiling water until just tender (about 10 minutes).

Warm the tomato sauce. Drain the pasta and mix in the sauce.

Serve sprinkled with a little chopped parsley.

Kidney Bean and Tomato Dinner

You can adapt this dish for older members of the family if desired by adding coriander and cumin powder together with some fresh and/or dried chilli.

1 small onion, chopped
sunflower oil for frying
1 clove garlic, crushed
1 tsp ground cumin (optional)
1 tsp ground coriander (optional)
1 400g (16oz) tin of tomatoes with juice
1 400g (16oz) tin red kidney beans, drained
fresh coriander leaves

Fry the onion in a little oil until just browning, then add the garlic (and the dried coriander and cumin if desired).

Whizz the tomatoes and their juice in a blender and pour over the onion and spice mixture and cook for a minute or two. Pour the kidney beans over the tomato mixture, cover and simmer gently for 20 minutes.

Before serving, sprinkle over the chopped coriander, purée, mash or chop as required by your baby.

For older babies, children and adults, serve with rice, chappati (see page 111) or slices of wholemeal pitta.

Bubble and Squeak Cakes

A great way to use up leftover cabbage, spring greens, Brussels sprouts or curly kale.

half a small onion, chopped (optional)
sunflower oil for frying
100 g (4 oz) mashed potatoes
100 g (4 oz) cooked cabbage, spring greens, Brussels sprouts or curly kale, chopped

In a frying pan, brown the onion in the oil. Cool and reserve.

Place the mashed potatoes and the chopped vegetables in a large bowl. Add the cooked onion and stir thoroughly to produce an even mixture. Pat the mixture into biscuit ring moulds (or any other shape you wish) and flatten down into 2.5 cm (1 inch) cakes. Fry gently in a large frying pan until golden. Remove the moulds and turn to brown on the other side. Alternatively, grill until golden on each side.

Red, Yellow and Green Rice

A feast for the eyes as well as the palate.

1 salad onion, chopped fine
sunflower oil for frying
a pinch of cumin seed
25 g (1 oz) long-grain rice, washed
50 ml (2 fl oz) vegetable stock or water
half a tomato, peeled, de-seeded and chopped
1 tsp tomato purée
1 tbsp frozen peas
1 tbsp frozen sweetcorn

Fry the onion in a little oil for a few minutes without browning. Add the cumin and cook for another minute or two.

Add the washed rice, stirring to coat each grain with the oil. Pour on the stock or water. Cover and cook very gently for about 5 minutes.

Add the tomato and tomato purée and cook for another 5 minutes.

Finally, stir in the peas and sweetcorn and cook for a further 5 minutes or until the rice is tender.

Serve with sticks of peeled cucumber and some Greek yoghurt or with fresh salad vegetables.

Kitcheri

When I was a child my mother often gave me kitcheri, a moist, aromatic mixture of rice and lentils flavoured with cinnamon, cloves and cardamom. Add peppercorns and cloves for older members of the family.

75 g (3 oz) long-grain rice
75 g (3 oz) red lentils
sunflower oil for frying
1 small onion, peeled and chopped fine
1 small clove of garlic, crushed
2.5 cm (1 inch) piece of cinnamon
2 cardamom pods
1 clove (optional)
3 peppercorns
300 ml (half a pint) of water

Combine the rice and lentils and wash in a colander under running water, then leave to soak for 20 minutes or so.

Heat the oil and fry the onion for 2 minutes. Add the garlic, cinnamon, cardamom, clove and peppercorns and fry for a further 2 or 3 minutes.

Drain the rice and lentil mixture, then add to the onion and garlic and sauté for a minute or two.

Add the water, cover and cook gently for 15 minutes until the rice is cooked.

Before serving, remove the cinnamon, cardamom, clove and peppercorns.

Serve with slices of tomato and peeled cucumber.

Veggie 'Tortillas'

This thick, Spanish omelet is packed with potatoes so it can be cut into thick wedges and served warm or cold. Add any cooked vegetables you like to this versatile recipe.

1 small onion, chopped
sunflower oil for frying
200 g (8 oz) diced potatoes
4 tbsp frozen peas
2 eggs, beaten
4 tbsp milk
chopped parsley

Fry the onion in the oil in a large frying pan until translucent (about 5 minutes). Turn down the heat and add the potatoes, frying very gently for about 10 minutes until cooked. Add the peas.

Beat the eggs and milk together and pour the mixture over the vegetables. Cook on a very low heat for about ten minutes. Finally, place the frying pan under a hot grill until set. Sprinkle on the parsley.

Cool, turn out onto a plate and cut into wedges.

Tomato Rice with Mushroom

1 small onion, chopped fine
sunflower oil for frying
25 g (1 oz) rice
1 200g (8 oz) tin of tomatoes with juice
50 g (2 oz) button mushrooms
1 tsp tomato paste
chopped fresh basil

Fry the onion in a little sunflower oil. Add the rice. Stir to coat well and cook for a minute or two until the rice becomes translucent.

Whizz the tomatoes in a blender until smooth and pour over the rice mixture.

Slice the mushrooms and add to the pan with the tomato paste. Cover and cook for about 15 minutes or until the rice is tender.

To finish, sprinkle with a little chopped basil.

Adjust the texture as necessary.

Courgette Risotto

Risotto is a traditional Italian dish and uses short-grain or arborio rice cooked in stock, which leads to a creamy consistency. You will get a creamier texture if the stock is added to the rice mixture slowly, one ladle-full at a time, although admittedly this is rather time consuming. If you wish, simply add all the liquid at once, but do remember to stir regularly.

1 small onion, chopped
1 small garlic clove, crushed
1 courgette, chopped
olive oil for frying

150 g (6 oz) arborio or short-grain rice
600 ml (1 pint) vegetable or chicken stock
75 ml (3 fl oz) apple juice

Sauté the onion, garlic and chopped courgette gently in a little olive oil in a heavy-bottomed pan for 4 minutes without browning. Add the rice and sauté for a minute or two, stirring to ensure that the rice becomes coated with the oil. Add the stock (one ladle-full at a time or all at once), then the apple juice. Simmer gently for about 20–25 minutes.

For older members of the family, serve with grated Parmesan rice and salad. For babies, serve with salad vegetables cut into finger-food size.

Cheesy Potatoes and Broccoli

100 g (4 oz) potato, peeled and chopped
50 g (2 oz) broccoli florets
125 ml (5 fl oz) white sauce
25 g (1 oz) grated Cheddar cheese

Boil the potatoes in a little fast boiling water in a covered pan until tender.

Cook the broccoli until tender (either boil, steam or cook in the microwave).

Make up the white sauce as on page 88, adding the cheese at the last minute and stirring in until smooth.

Mix together the potato and the broccoli and pour on the cheese sauce, adding a little of the cooking water from the broccoli if necessary.

Purée or chop as necessary. For older babies, children (or adults) pour into a serving dish and sprinkle with some more grated cheese. Grill until bubbling.

Breads

Chappati

An unleavened Indian bread.

> 50 g (2 oz) wholemeal flour
> 50 g (2 oz) plain flour
> 1 tbsp sunflower oil
> approximately 100 ml (4 fl oz) water
> more flour as needed
> butter or sunflower oil as needed

Mix together the two types of flour. Add the oil. Gradually add the water and mix for 4 or 5 minutes, until the dough has gathered into a ball. Cover and leave in the fridge for half an hour.

Using a knife, cut the dough into two, then four, then eight pieces. Roll each piece into a ball and roll out on a floured surface into a thin round. Cook on a lightly greased griddle; when the blisters appear, press down using a fish slice. Turn the chappati over to cook the other side. Brush with a little butter or sunflower oil.

Chappatis go well with Indian or North African dishes.

Potato and Pumpkin Damper

'Damper' is a type of bread made without yeast which the first immigrants to Australia used to make to sustain them when working long days in the bush. It is designed to be eaten soon after cooking (or else it will dry out rapidly), but can be frozen. Try this recipe using pumpkin, a favourite Australian vegetable.

1 tsp sunflower margarine or butter
200 g (8 oz) flour, sifted
75 g (3 oz) baked pumpkin, mashed
25 g (1 oz) mashed potatoes
2 tsp chives, snipped
water
additional flour as needed

Rub the margarine or butter into the sifted flour and stir in the pumpkin, potatoes and chives. Add water to form a sticky dough (take care not to add too much water too quickly so that the mixture becomes too wet).

Place on a floured surface and knead gently. Place in a hot oven (Gas Mark 6/200°C/400°F) for about 10 minutes. Reduce the heat slightly and continue to bake for a further 10 to 15 minutes.

Serve with casseroles or soups.

Cheesy Muffins

100 g (4 oz) flour, sifted
pinch of salt
1 tsp baking powder
100 ml (4 fl oz) milk or buttermilk
1 egg
1 tbsp sunflower oil
100 g (4 oz) finely grated Cheddar or Cheshire cheese

Sieve the flour, salt and baking powder in a large bowl.

In a separate bowl, beat together the milk, oil and egg. Make a well in centre of flour mixture and pour in the milk mixture. Stir well.

Sprinkle over the cheese and fold in. Pour into cake papers and bake in a moderate oven (Gas Mark 4/180°C/350°F) for 30 minutes.

Homemade Rusks

Hard finger-foods can help ease sore gums, but shop-bought rusks can contain large amounts of sugar, so do read the labels. You can easily make your own rusks at home – by slow baking bread.

Cut a thick slice of bread into easy-to-hold fingers and bake in the oven (Gas Mark 4/180°C/350°F) for about 20 minutes.

VARIATION
Brush the bread with honey or yeast extract (Marmite) diluted 50:50 with water before baking.

French Toast

1 egg
2 tbsp milk
1 slice bread (wholemeal or white)
sunflower margarine for frying

Whisk together the egg and the milk. Soak the bread in the milk-and-egg mixture, turning the bread once. Fry until brown on both sides.

VARIATIONS
Spread a tiny scrape of yeast extract on the bread before dipping into the egg mixture and frying.

Add a pinch of cinnamon to the egg mixture.

Cut the bread into two and sprinkle over a little grated cheese, then sandwich the bread together and warm through once more in the frying pan.

Polenta with Oregano

This Italian cornmeal makes the ideal accompaniment to stews and casseroles, or serve it to your baby cut into strips as a finger-food with a dip (see below for dip recipes).

75 g (3 oz) polenta
1 tsp fresh oregano
1 tbsp sunflower margarine or butter

Cook the polenta according to the instructions on the packet, stirring in the oregano and the butter or margarine as it starts to thicken together.

For older members of the family, stir in a little grated Parmesan cheese.

Cool and cut into wedges or fingers and grill until golden, turning once.

Dips

Cheesy Dip with Mint, Chives and Cucumber

50 g (2 oz) cream cheese
3 tbsp Greek yoghurt
2 tsp grated Cheddar cheese
1 tsp chopped mint
1 tsp snipped chives
quarter of a cucumber, peeled and grated

Mix the cream cheese and yoghurt in a large bowl and beat well. Fold in the cheese, mint, chives and cucumber.

Serve with crunchy vegetable sticks, halved baby tomatoes, pieces of fruit such as pear and apple, breadsticks and unsalted crackers.

Tzaziki

A Middle Eastern yoghurt dip made with cucumber. Try offering unsalted crackers or slices of toasted wholemeal pitta bread to dip and dunk.

1 cucumber
2 tbsp thick unsweetened yoghurt
fresh mint, chopped

Wash, peel and grate the cucumber then squeeze out the excess liquid with your hands. Spoon the yoghurt into a small bowl and add the cucumber to it. Sprinkle over the chopped mint, stir and serve.

This recipe does not freeze well.

Puddings

Mango Cream

Mango is a delicious, sweet and fragrant fruit. Choose a fruit that is firm but will yield gently when pressed at the stalk end.

> 1 small ripe mango
> cooked baby rice

Peel the mango with a sharp knife. Push the skin outwards and scoop out the flesh.

Purée or mash the mango and stir into the baby rice.

Stewed Rhubarb with Orange Custard

FOR THE RHUBARB

Choose young pink stems for the sweetest taste. Trim both ends and chop into equal-sized pieces. Add just a little boiling water, but not so much that it covers the fruit. Bring to the boil, cover and simmer for about 10 minutes. Add a pinch of ground ginger if you wish. Add a little muscovado sugar to taste while still warm and set aside.

FOR THE CUSTARD

To make about 300 ml (half a pint) of custard.

> 2 eggs
> 1 tsp runny honey
> 300 ml (half a pint) of milk
> 1 tsp grated orange rind

In a large bowl, whisk together the eggs, honey and 4 tbsp of the milk. Place the bowl over a large pan of gently simmering water and whisk in the rest of the milk slowly. Continue to whisk the custard and cook until the mixture thickens. Stir in the orange rind.

Serve warm or cold with the cooked rhubarb (or any other stewed fruit).

Apple and Kiwi Yoghurt

Rich and tangy, kiwi fruits are also rich in vitamin C. Mixing it with apple and yoghurt gives it a less sharp, more creamy taste.

> 1 eating apple, peeled, cored and chopped
> 1 ripe kiwi fruit, peeled and chopped
> 1 tbsp Greek yoghurt

Cook and purée the apple in the usual way and set aside.

Chop the kiwi fruit (if your baby is very young, you may want to push the kiwi fruit through a sieve to remove the seeds). Mix with the apple mixture. Stir in the yoghurt.

Rice Pudding

> 50 g (2 oz) pudding rice
> 600 ml (1 pint) milk
> 1 tbsp sugar

Put the rice in a heavy-bottomed pan and add the milk and the sugar. Bring to the boil, then lower the heat and simmer gently for 30 minutes, stirring occasionally.

Fragrant Rice Pudding with Orange and Cardamom

100 g (2 oz) pudding rice
600 ml (1 pint) milk
1 cardamom pod
1 tbsp sultanas
1 tsp grated orange rind
1 tbsp fresh orange juice or unsweetened orange juice

Put the rice in a heavy-bottomed pan and add the milk, cardamom pod and sultanas. Bring to the boil, then lower to simmering heat, stirring occasionally, for about 30 minutes or so. Take off the heat and stir in the orange rind and juice and cook for another 5 minutes.

Fruity Porridge

Liven up ordinary porridge by adding fruit purée to made-up porridge. Try banana or stewed apple instead of apricot, or any other fruit you prefer.

15 g (½ ounce) rolled oats
50 ml (2 fl oz) full-fat cows' milk or your baby's usual milk
half a tin of apricots, drained

Over a low heat, simmer the oats and milk for about 5 minutes. Cool, then stir in the puréed apricot or your chosen fruit.

Homemade Yoghurt

Making homemade yoghurt is not difficult – this method has been used for centuries on the Indian subcontinent.

2 tsp shop-bought natural bio-yoghurt
600 ml (1 pint) full-fat milk

Pour the milk into a large pan and bring to the boil. Take off the heat as the milk begins to rise. Cool the pan slightly by dipping it into a sink of cold water, then pour it into a large bowl. Stir in the bought yoghurt, cover and place in a cool oven (the lowest setting your oven will go). Allow to set overnight.

Homemade Strawberry Yoghurt

4 ripe strawberries
homemade or Greek yoghurt
1 tsp unsweetened orange juice

Wash the fruit and pass through a sieve to remove the hard pips. Combine with the yoghurt and add the orange juice.

Eccles Cakes

Try these delicious pastries for a special treat which originated in Lancashire.

1 packet frozen puff pastry, defrosted
flour as needed
25 g (1 oz) butter
125 g (5 oz) currants
25 g (1 oz) mixed peel
milk for brushing

Roll out the pastry on a lightly floured surface and cut out 12 rounds using pastry cutters or a small glass. Melt the butter and pour over the fruit. Divide the fruit and peel between the rounds. Then, using a pastry brush, dampen edges with water and bring them together.

Turn the cakes over, brush with a little milk and, using a sharp knife, cut out a cross shape on the top of each cake.

Place on a baking tray and bake in a hot oven (Gas Mark 7/220°C/425°F) for 15 to 20 minutes or until golden brown.

Freeze any remaining cakes.

Peach Melba

A variation of an old favourite.

    half a peach (fresh or tinned)
    1 tbsp fresh or tinned raspberries
    3 tbsp Greek yoghurt

Peel the peach and remove the stone. Purée. Pass the raspberries through a sieve to remove the pips. Mix together the fruit purées and then stir in the Greek yoghurt.

You can replace the Greek yoghurt with a scoop of vanilla ice cream if you wish.

Banana Smoothie

A delicious drink that doubles up as a liquid pudding!

    half a ripe banana, chopped
    50 ml (2 fl oz) your baby's usual milk
    1 scoop vanilla ice cream

Place all the ingredients in an electric blender and whizz until mixed and frothy. Serve immediately.

This recipe does not freeze well.

Autumn Pudding

Similar to summer pudding, this delicious dessert makes use of the succulent fruits that are abundant in the autumn and winter months. If you wish, you can use summer fruits. Do make sure that you remove any difficult to digest berry pips first by sieving.

> 500 g (1 lb) mixed autumn fruit (apples, blackberries, plums and pears)
> 4 tbsp water
> about 5 slices bread, crusts removed
> 1 tbsp brown sugar

Wash the fruit, removing the skins, pips/stones and seeds. Place in a large pan. Add water, cover and simmer for about 10 minutes or until the fruit is cooked. Allow to cool slightly.

Cut a round of bread to fit the base of a 1-pint pudding basin. Slice the remaining bread into fingers and use it to line the pudding bowl, making sure you do not leave any gaps. Spoon the fruit mixture into the bowl on top of the bread and until just under the rim, reserving any extra juice. Use the remaining bread to make a lid for the pudding. Cover with foil and then a plate. Place a weight on top and allow to cool. Place in the fridge overnight.

To loosen the pudding, run a knife around the edges and turn onto a plate. Pour over any remaining liquid to moisten the pudding.

11

---

9 to 12 Months

Once your baby is nine months of age, she will probably have some teeth – it is important to gently encourage your baby to progress to minced or chopped foods. Finger-foods are important too, as these will help encourage self-feeding and hone hand–eye coordination. Also, harder finger-foods can help to ease the discomfort of teething (there are some suggestions later in this chapter).

Remember that the recipes in Chapter 10 are still appropriate for your growing baby (and for the rest of the family!).

Every Morning Muesli

25 g (1 oz) fine oatmeal
1 tsp each prunes, peaches and raisins, soaked and sieved to remove the tough skins
50 ml (2 fl oz) unsweetened apple juice
mango, paw paw or banana to serve
milk or yoghurt to serve

Mix the oats and sieved prunes, peaches and raisins together in a bowl. Add the apple juice. Cover and keep in the fridge overnight.

Just before serving, stir in a little chopped mango or paw paw and banana and pour on the cold fresh milk or a dollop of yoghurt. Adjust the consistency as required.

Chicken Meals

Indian Chicken with Lime

This mild and aromatic dish is quick and delicious and is sure to be a winner with all the family. For adults, you can use a hot tandoori paste and add chopped fresh green chilli to taste at the marinade stage.

    1 free-range chicken breast
    $\frac{1}{2}$ to 1 tsp mild Tandoori paste (available from supermarkets)
    1 200 g (8 oz) carton Greek or natural yoghurt
    1 tsp fresh lime juice

Cut the chicken into strips and place in a mixing bowl.

Mix the mild Tandoori paste with the yoghurt and the fresh lime juice. Cover and leave in the fridge overnight.

Place in a heavy-bottomed pan and simmer for 20 minutes on a moderate heat until cooked right through.

Serve with boiled rice or toasted pitta bread and salad.

Sweet and Sour Chicken with Mango

    sunflower oil for frying
    1 free-range chicken breast

25 ml (1 fl oz) apple juice
1 tbsp low-salt soy sauce
1 tsp brown sugar
50 g (2 oz) carrots
¼ green pepper
1 200 g (8 oz) tin tomatoes
½ ripe mango, diced
50 g (2 oz) beansprouts

Sauté the chicken in a large casserole or wok. Add the apple juice, soy sauce and sugar and stir well.

Slice the carrots and cut the pepper into strips and add to the casserole dish along with the tomatoes. Cover and cook for 25 minutes on a medium heat.

Add the chopped mango and beansprouts and continue cooking for another 5 minutes. Adjust the consistency as required.

Serve with rice.

Chicken, Banana and Apple Curry

This recipe uses mild curry powder. You can use hot curry powder for adults.

sunflower oil for frying
1 small onion, chopped
1 tsp ground cumin
1 tsp mild curry powder
1 free-range chicken breast
1 200 g (8 oz) tin tomatoes
1 eating apple, peeled, cored and chopped
1 small banana

Sauté the onion, cumin and curry powder in a little hot sunflower oil until the onion is soft. Add the chicken pieces and brown slightly.

Whizz the tomatoes in a blender until smooth, add to the chicken mixture, cover and simmer for 5 minutes.

Add the chopped apple and sliced banana and cook for a further 10 minutes.

Mash or adjust the consistency as required.

Serve with boiled rice, chappati or toasted wholemeal pitta.

Singapore Noodles with Chicken

For older members of the family and for a more authentic version, add a dash of sherry, chopped chilli and prawns during the cooking process.

50 g (2 oz) noodles
groundnut or sunflower oil for frying
1 spring onion, chopped fine
$^1/_2$ clove of garlic, crushed
1 tsp grated ginger
50 g (2 oz) cooked chicken, chopped
2 button mushrooms, sliced
1 tsp low–salt soy sauce
1 tsp apple juice
150 ml ($^1/_4$ pint) water or chicken stock

Cook the noodles in plenty of boiling water until tender. Drain and reserve.

Fry the onion, garlic and ginger in a large frying pan or wok until translucent (take care not to allow the ginger to burn). Add to this the chicken, mushrooms and the drained noodles. Stir well to ensure all the ingredients are coated. Cook for another 2 or 3 minutes before adding the soy sauce, apple juice and stock. Stir in well. Cover and simmer very gently for 5 minutes.

Grated Potato Cakes with Chicken and Vegetables

A treat for all the family and a great way to use up leftover cooked chicken.

    100 g (4 oz) of potatoes
    1 egg, beaten
    80 ml (3 fl oz) milk
    50 g (2 oz) flour
    100 g (4 oz) cooked chicken, chopped into small pieces
    2 tbsp frozen peas
    2 tbsp frozen sweetcorn
    1 tbsp chopped chives or parsley

Peel and grate the potatoes and cook in a little boiling water in the microwave. Squeeze out the extra liquid and drain on kitchen paper.

Whisk the egg together with the milk. Add the flour slowly, whisking to avoid any lumps. Add the chicken, peas and sweetcorn and stir, adding more milk if necessary to produce a sloppy mixture. Stir in the chives and parsley.

Using a metal biscuit cutter placed in a frying pan with some oil, pour a spoonful of the mixture into the shape and cook over a gentle heat until the cakes are golden brown, turning once.

Meat Meals

Beef

Corned Beef Hash

An old family favourite, you can make this dish from the ingredients in your larder. It only takes about 20 minutes to cook and is a good source of iron.

250 g (9 oz) potatoes, peeled and diced
sunflower oil for frying
1 small onion, peeled and chopped
1 200 g (8 oz) tin baked beans
1 200 g (8 oz) tin corned beef, diced
50 g (2 oz) Cheddar cheese, grated
1 tbsp chopped parsley

Cook the potatoes in a little boiling water in a covered pan for about 10 minutes.

Fry the onion in a little sunflower oil until soft, then add the drained potatoes, the baked beans, the corned beef and most of the cheese. Sprinkle over the parsley and mix thoroughly. Place in an oven-proof dish. Cook in a moderate oven (Gas Mark 5/190°C/375°F) for 10 minutes.

Just before serving, add a little more grated cheese and place under a hot grill for a few minutes until golden and bubbling.

Spinach Beef with Tomato

150 g (6 oz) beef, cut into strips
flour for coating
olive oil for frying
1 small onion
$^1/_2$ clove garlic, crushed
pinch cumin powder
pinch coriander powder
1 200 g (8 oz) tin tomatoes, whizzed in the blender
50 g (2 oz) spinach, stalks removed
Greek yoghurt or fromage frais to serve

Put the strips of beef in a clean plastic bag with a little flour, close and shake until coated.

Fry the onion, then add the garlic and the coated beef and cook for about 5 minutes.

Add the cumin, coriander and tomatoes; cover and cook for another 5 minutes.

Add the spinach leaves and cook for a further 3 or 4 minutes.

Remove from heat and stir in the Greek yoghurt or fromage frais.

Serve with pasta or rice and vegetables.

Lamb

Lamb Meatballs with Cinnamon, Coconut and Cardamom

These meatballs are both aromatic and sweet due to the addition of cardamom, coconut and tomato purée.

200 g (8 oz) lean minced lamb
1 tbsp desiccated coconut

1 tsp cardamom powder
pinch cinnamon powder
3 tbsp tomato purée
1 tbsp chopped fresh mint
1 egg, beaten
flour for coating
sunflower oil for frying

Place the meat in a large bowl and add the coconut, cardamom, cinnamon and tomato purée. Mix together. Pour over the beaten egg and mix well.

Divide the mixture into 16 small balls and roll each ball in a plate of flour.

Heat the oil in a frying pan on a moderate heat and fry each meatball until golden, turning once.

Serve with tomato sauce or tomato rice and salad vegetables, or dunk into Greek yoghurt with grated cucumber.

Greek Moussaka

This classic Greek dish is a mixture of minced lamb and aubergines topped with a cheesy sauce. For a non-meat treat, simply replace the lamb with more aubergine.

olive oil for frying
half an aubergine, sliced
100 g (4 oz) potatoes, peeled and sliced
1 small onion, chopped
100 g (4 oz) lean lamb mince
1 200 g (8 oz) tin tomatoes, whizzed in a blender
2 tsp tomato purée
flat leaf parsley, chopped

1 small egg, beaten
5 tbsp Greek yoghurt
25 g (1 oz) grated Gruyere cheese

Brush the slices of aubergine and grill for 5 minutes or until browned under a medium grill, then turn and brown the other side. Set aside.

Cook the potatoes in a covered pan in a little boiling water until tender (about 6–8 minutes). Drain and set aside

Fry the onion in a little olive oil for 4 or 5 minutes until browned and then add the minced lamb. Cook for another few minutes, then add the tomatoes, the tomato purée and the parsley. Cover and simmer for 15 to 20 minutes.

Spoon half of the meat in an ovenproof dish, add a layer of the aubergine, then repeat with alternate layers of meat and aubergine. Top with a layer of potatoes.

Whisk the egg and beat in the Greek yoghurt. Pour the yoghurt mixture over the casserole. Sprinkle on the cheese. Bake in a moderate oven (Gas Mark 4/180°C/350°F) for 30 minutes until golden and bubbling.

Serve with salad and bread.

Moroccan Lamb with Beans

Lightly spiced, this lamb dish is very tender. Green beans are a traditional accompaniment to lamb.

sunflower oil for frying
50 g (2 oz) cubed lamb
1 salad onion, chopped
½ tsp ground cumin
½ tsp ground cinnamon
100 ml (4 fl oz) vegetable or chicken stock

1 chopped tomato, skinned, deseeded and chopped
$\frac{1}{2}$ tsp tomato purée
50 g (2 oz) frozen green beans
$\frac{1}{2}$ tsp each flat leaf parsley and mint, chopped

Fry the lamb over a low heat until just browning, then add the onion, cumin and coriander and cook gently for another 5 minutes. Pour over the stock, add the tomato and tomato purée and turn down the heat. Simmer gently for 20 minutes.

Add the beans and simmer for another 10 minutes or so until the meat is tender. Sprinkle with the parsley and mint.

Serve with bread, rice or couscous and tomato salad.

Mini Meatballs with Pasta Shapes

Make these mini meatballs small enough for your baby to pick up and use as finger-foods, or bigger for older members of the family.

100 g (4 oz) minced lamb (or beef)
half a small onion, chopped
1 tbsp chopped fresh basil
1 tbsp chopped fresh parsley

To make the meatballs, simply place all the ingredients into a large bowl and mix well, or, alternatively, whizz in a food processor for a minute or two until well mixed. Divide and shape into 5 large or 15 small meatballs. Cover and keep in the fridge.

TO MAKE THE SAUCE
olive oil for frying
1 small onion
1 clove garlic, crushed

1 400 g (16 oz) tin tomatoes, blended in a food processor
1 tbsp tomato paste
100 ml (4 fl oz) chicken stock

Fry the onion and garlic in a little olive oil in a large pan until soft (about 5 minutes). Add the tomatoes, tomato paste and chicken stock; stir well. Bring to simmering point, then add the meatballs. Cover and simmer very gently for 30 minutes, ensuring that the meatballs are cooked all the way through.

75 g (3 oz) pasta shapes, cooked
parsley and mint to serve

Cook the pasta according to the directions on the packet.

Pour the meatball and tomato mixture over the warm, cooked pasta. Sprinkle with chopped parsley and fresh basil.

Fish Meals

Fish Pie with Egg and Tomato

250 g (8 oz) skinless haddock fillets
1 boiled egg
1 tomato, deseeded and chopped (for older babies and children, simply cut into quarters)
50 g (2 oz) frozen peas
250 g (8 oz) potatoes
milk and butter or margarine as needed

FOR THE CHEESE SAUCE

    25 g (1 oz) flour

    25 g (1 oz) sunflower margarine or butter

    300 ml ('/2 pint) milk

    50 g (2 oz) medium matured Cheddar cheese

Place the fish between two plates and steam or microwave until just tender. Flake the fish and remove any bones; place in a serving dish.

For the cheese sauce, make the white sauce in the usual way (see page 88). Stir in most of the grated cheese, reserving a little.

Add the egg, tomato and peas to the cheese sauce. Pour the sauce over the fish.

Peel and wash the potatoes and cut into small pieces. Cook in a little fast boiling water in a covered pan until tender (about 5 minutes). Drain and mash with a little milk and margarine or butter. Pile on top of the fish and sprinkle over the reserved grated cheese. Place in a moderate oven (Gas Mark 4/180°C/350°F) and cook for 20 minutes.

Serve with vegetables such as carrots, broccoli and/or sweetcorn.

Fish Chowder

A chowder is a hearty soup thickened with potatoes.

    sunflower oil for frying

    1 small onion

    50 g (2 oz) potatoes, diced

    half a carrot, peeled and cut into discs

    600 ml (1 pint) vegetable or fish stock

    100 g (4 oz) unsmoked cod or haddock fillet

    1 tbsp frozen peas

    1 tbsp frozen corn

Fry the onion in a casserole. Add the potatoes and carrot and pour over the stock. Cover and simmer gently for about 15 minutes.

Add the fish and simmer for another 5 minutes.

Add the peas and sweetcorn and cook for a further 5 minutes.

Mash or purée if necessary; serve with bread to dunk.

Cheesy Fish Shapes

Try and use a fish cutter to give these fish cakes visual appeal, or simply shape into flat rounds.

6 oz (150 g) skinned white fish such as haddock or coley
2 oz (50 g) frozen peas, defrosted
1 oz (25 g) Cheshire cheese, grated
1 egg, beaten
15 g (1 tbsp) flour
flour for dusting
sunflower oil for frying

Chop the fish and whizz in a food processor for a minute or two. Mix this fish purée with the peas and cheese. Add the beaten egg and the flour and mix well (you may want to add a little more flour if the mixture is too sloppy).

Divide the mixture into 8 portions. With floured hands, shape fish cakes into balls or use small fish cutters and flatten down gently.

Fry in a little sunflower oil until golden, turning once.

Alternatively, grill the fish cakes: brush with a little oil and grill under a moderate heat for 4–5 minutes or until golden, turning once.

Serve with baked beans and mashed potatoes.

Vegetable Meals

Couscous with Courgette, Pepper and Mushrooms

Couscous are grains of semolina that have been coated with wheat flour. Couscous is very popular in North Africa and can be used to accompany poultry, meat or vegetable dishes, or in stews or as a salad with vegetables and fresh herbs.

1 small courgette, washed and sliced
1 red pepper, deseeded and sliced
4 button mushrooms, sliced
1 200 g (8 oz) tin tomatoes, blended in the food processor
olive oil
75 g (3 oz) couscous
80 ml (3 fl oz) water or vegetable stock
1 tbsp flat leaf parsley, chopped

Sauté the courgette, pepper, mushrooms and tomatoes in a little olive oil for 4 or 5 minutes until cooked. Set aside.

Pour the couscous into a pan filled with 3 fl oz boiling water or stock. Bring down the heat to simmering, cover and cook for about 3 minutes or until the couscous has absorbed the fluid and can be 'fluffed' with a fork.

Mix the vegetables with the couscous and serve sprinkled with the parsley.

Caribbean Rice 'n' Peas

The peas in this West Indian dish are actually beans. For older children and adults, you can add hot flavourings like chopped chilli pepper.

sunflower oil for frying
1 small onion, chopped
100 g (4 oz) minced pork
150 g (6 oz) long-grain rice
600 ml (1 pint) chicken or vegetable stock
1 200 g (8 oz) tin red kidney beans, drained
50 g (1 oz) creamed coconut
1 tbsp fresh coriander, chopped

Fry the onion in a little sunflower oil with the pork for about 5 minutes.

Wash the rice in a little water, drain and add to the onions. Stir and cook for another 5 minutes.

Add the stock, cover and simmer for 5 minutes. Add the drained beans, the creamed coconut and a little more stock or water if the mixture looks dry. Cook for another 10 minutes. Sprinkle on the coriander.

Serve with salad vegetables.

Courgette Lasagne

sunflower onion for frying
1 small onion, chopped
1 clove of garlic, crushed
500 g (1 lb) courgettes
1 400 g (16 oz) tin tomatoes, blended until smooth in a liquidizer
2 tsp tomato purée
300 ml (½ pint) vegetable stock
25 g (1 oz) flour
50 ml (2 oz) water
200 ml (7 fl oz) white sauce
75 g (3 oz) Gruyere cheese, grated
lasagne sheets

Fry the onion and the garlic in the sunflower oil. After a few minutes, add the sliced courgettes and cook for another 5 minutes or until tender.

Add the tomatoes, tomato purée and stock.

Sprinkle the flour in a little cold water and mix to make a smooth paste. Stir into the courgette mixture, mixing well to avoid lumps. Cover and simmer for 20 minutes.

Prepare the white sauce (see page 88), stirring in most of the grated cheese. Set by.

Ladle the courgette mixture into a large oven-proof dish and cover with a layer of the lasagna sheets. Alternate layers of courgette and lasagna twice more, finishing with a layer of lasagne.

Pour the cheese sauce over the lasagne carefully so that all the pasta is covered. Sprinkle with the remaining cheese. Bake in a moderate oven (Gas Mark 5/190°C/375°F) for 20 minutes until golden and bubbling.

Falafels

Falafels are Middle Eastern meat-free burgers made with chick peas. For older children and adults, serve in pitta pockets loaded with slices of tomato, cucumber and chopped parsley and coriander. And for those adults who can take it, drizzle with a little chilli sauce.

100 g (4 oz) tinned or cooked chick peas, drained
1 tbsp flat leaf parsley, chopped fine
2 tsp fresh lemon juice
3 tbsp fresh coriander leaves, chopped fine
1 clove garlic, crushed
1 tsp ground cumin
1 tbsp flour
oil for frying

Mix the first seven ingredients in a blender and whizz until combined and smooth.

With slightly wet hands, divide into 15 to 20 portions and flatten with your hands to produce small, burger shapes. Fry in the hot oil, taking care not to overcrowd the pan. Turn once. Cook until golden brown, then drain.

Serve warm with salad and pitta bread spread with hummus (see page 140), or offer them with a yoghurt dip.

Bread

Banana Loaf

This makes a tasty snack, dessert or accompaniment with soups or salads.

    100 g (4 oz) butter
    100 g (4 oz) brown sugar
    1 egg
    200 g (8 oz) plain flour
    100 g (4 oz) self-raising flour
    1 tsp baking soda
    250 g (10 oz) mashed ripe bananas (2 large or 3 small)
    50 ml (2 fl oz) plain yoghurt

Mix the butter and sugar together until light and creamy. Beat in the egg.

In another bowl, sift together the flour and baking soda.

In a third bowl, combine the bananas and yoghurt, stirring just enough to mix.

Add dry ingredients alternately with the banana mixture to the butter/sugar, stirring just enough to combine well.

Turn into an oiled loaf pan. Bake (Gas Mark 5/190°C/375°F) for 50 to 60 minutes or until done.

Dips

Tomato and Cucumber Raita

The perfect dip, this raita can be eaten with raw vegetable sticks or breadsticks, pitta or chappati, or used as a traditional accompaniment to savoury Indian dishes. For a bigger 'bite' which older family members will love, add a little garam masal and some chilli powder.

1 200 g (8 oz) carton plain yoghurt
pinch ground cumin seeds
squeeze of lemon juice
1 tomato, peeled, deseeded and chopped
1 5 cm (2 inch) piece of cucumber, peeled and grated
1 tsp fresh coriander, chopped

Pour the yoghurt into a bowl, stir in the cumin and the lemon juice. Add the tomato and cucumber and sprinkle over the coriander.

Guacamole

An ideal dip for your baby to dunk which older children and adults will enjoy, too. You can add chopped red onion, garlic and chopped fresh chillis to taste for older members of the family. Serve soon after preparing or the avocado will discolour.

1 ripe avocado, peeled and stone removed
juice of half a lemon
1 ripe tomato, peeled, de-seeded and chopped

Combine all ingredients and whizz in a liquidizer or mash until smooth.

Serve with bread, breadsticks or warm pitta bread.

Hummus

Easy to make and delicious, try this Middle Eastern dip with sticks of vegetables, breadsticks, unsalted crackers or toasted pitta pieces.

1 400 g (16 oz) tin chick peas, drained
2 tbsp olive oil
1 tsp dried cumin
2 tsp tahini (sesame seed paste)
1 garlic clove, crushed
2 tbsp fresh lemon juice

Place all the ingredients in a food processor and whizz until smooth (older children and adults may prefer a slightly coarser version).

Serve with tomato wedges and strips of toasted pitta bread or breadsticks, or in a sandwich with grated carrot for older children.

Puddings

Baked Apple

   1 ripe eating apple, cored
   1 tsp sultanas or raisins
   sunflower margarine or butter
   100 ml (4 fl oz) unsweetened apple juice

Core the apple and slit the skin. Place on a baking dish. Stuff the dried fruits inside the apple, dab the margarine or butter over the top. Pour over the apple juice.

Cook in the oven (Gas Mark 5/190°C/375°F) for 30 to 40 minutes until brown and sizzling.

Serve with custard.

For a very young baby, peel off the skin and purée the apple and dried fruit.

Thai Coconut Rice

   25 g (1 oz) pudding rice
   1 level tbsp sugar (or to taste)
   150 ml (¼ pint) milk
   150 ml (¼ pint) coconut milk

Wash and drain the rice. Place in a 1-pint ovenproof dish. Mix the sugar (if using) with the milk and coconut milk and pour over the rice. Mix well.

Place in a preheated oven (Gas Mark 2/150°C/300°F) for about 1 hour.

Serve warm or cold.

Banana Bake with Vanilla

Fast and fantastic, baking the banana will bring out its naturally sweet flavour.

> a ripe banana
> 50 ml (2 fl oz) fresh orange juice
> 1 vanilla pod

Peel and slice the banana lengthwise and place in a small oven-proof dish. Pour over the orange juice. Add the vanilla pod and bake in a moderate oven (Gas Mark 4/180°C/350°F) for 10–15 minutes.

Serve with Greek yoghurt or custard.

Cinnamon Toast with Mango

A fruity twist for a teatime treat.

> 2 slices raisin bread
> butter or margarine
> ½ tsp cinnamon
> a quarter of a ripe mango, mashed
> Greek yoghurt

Toast the bread.

Melt a little butter or margarine and sprinkle in the cinnamon. Pour this mixture over one slice of the toast.

Spread the mango over this and top with a little Greek yoghurt. Cover with the other slice of toasted raisin bread.

Banana, Cinnamon and Orange Rice Pudding

    half a small banana
    100 g (4 oz) rice pudding (see page 117)
    2 tbsp fresh orange juice
    1 tsp finely grated orange rind
    ¼ tsp cinnamon

Slice the banana and place in a microwave on medium heat for 30 seconds. Place into an ovenproof dish. Top with the rice pudding and the juice.

Mix together the orange rind and cinnamon and sprinkle over the banana/rice mixture. Bake in a moderate oven (Gas Mark 4/180°C/350°F) for 10 minutes until warmed through.

Serve hot or cold.

Raspberry and Passion Fruit Sauce

This rich, tangy sauce takes just a few minutes to prepare and is great drizzled over Greek yoghurt, fromage frais or milk puddings.

    1 400 g (16 oz) tin raspberries in fruit juice
    1 ripe passion fruit
    juice of half an orange

Pour the raspberries and juice into a large sieve and, with the back of a spoon, purée the fruit into a large bowl.

Cut the passion fruit into halves and do the same. Stir in the orange juice.

Tropical Fruit Salad

1 passion fruit
50 ml (2 fl oz) fresh unsweetened pineapple juice
half a fresh pineapple
half a mango, cut into cubes
1 slice cantaloupe melon, peeled and diced
10 green grapes, deseeded and peeled if necessary
half a banana, cut into discs
1 tsp chopped mint

Cut the passion fruit in two, scrape out the seeds with a spoon and place in a sieve. Sieve the seeds and reserve the liquid.

Mix the passion fruit liquid with the pineapple juice. Set aside.

Prepare the pineapple by trimming and cutting away the skin together with any hard pits and the centre circle, which can be a little tough. Cut the pineapple into manageable chunks. Place in a large serving dish.

Next, prepare the mango and add to the pineapple.

Add the melon, grapes (skins removed if necessary) and banana.

Pour over the pineapple and passion fruit mixture and sprinkle with the chopped mint.

The fruits in this salad may be a little sharp, so soften the flavour by serving with some fromage frais or yoghurt.

Bread and Butter Pudding with Apricots

A fruity twist to an old family favourite.

3 slices white bread
50 g (2 oz) butter or sunflower margarine
2 tinned apricot halves, drained and puréed

75 g (3 oz) sultanas
2 eggs, beaten
300 ml ($\frac{1}{2}$ pint) milk
vanilla essence
50 g (2 oz) sugar (or less if desired)

Remove crusts from the bread and spread with butter or margarine and a layer of puréed apricot.

Place a layer of the bread on the bottom of a small, shallow pie dish (butter side up). Sprinkle with sultanas.

Continue alternating layers of bread and sultanas, finishing with a layer of bread on the top (apricot and butter side down).

Whisk together the eggs, milk, vanilla essence and sugar; strain. Pour the milk mixture over the bread and butter and bake in a moderate oven (Gas Mark 4/180°C/350°F).

Serve with a dollop of natural yoghurt.

Snacks and Light Meal Ideas

Finally, here are some tempting snack ideas good for any time of day:

- ❏ plain cereal – puffed rice, porridge or corn flakes
- ❏ sandwiches, rolls or pitta bread made with fish, meat, egg, or cheese
- ❏ toast or bread with smooth peanut butter
- ❏ sliced fruit or vegetables
- ❏ unsweetened yoghurt with chopped or puréed fruit
- ❏ chopped hard boiled egg and watercress
- ❏ breadsticks
- ❏ hummus and grated carrot in toasted pitta parcels
- ❏ soft, cooked beans in tomato sauce

Useful Addresses

The National Childbirth Trust

Alexandra House
Oldham Terrace
London W3 6NH
0181 992 8637

The Coeliac Society

PO Box 220
High Wycombe
Bucks HP11 2HY

Cystic Fibrosis Research Trust

Alexandra House
5 Blyth Road
Bromley
Kent BR1 3RS

The Vegetarian Society

Parkdale
Dunham Road
Altrincham
Cheshire WA14 4QG

The Vegan Society

Donald Watson House
7 Battle Road
St Leonard's-on-Sea
East Sussex TN37 7AA
01424 427 393

British Allergy Foundation

Deepdene House
30 Bellegrove Road
Welling
Kent DA16 3PY
0181 303 8525

National Asthma Campaign

Providence House
Providence Place
London N1 0NT

Soil Association

Bristol House
40–56 Victoria Street
Bristol BS1 6BY
0117 929 0661

Index

additives 28, 38
adult drinks 29
allergies 32–3, 34–7
antioxidants 9

baby rice 67
barley 28
bottlefeeding 22–5, 39, 47
bottles, cleaning 23–4
breastfeeding 16–20, 47, 58
breastmilk 15–16

calcium 11, 16–17
calendars see weaning
    calendars
calories 3
canned foods 65
carbohydrates 3, 5
carbonated drinks 30
cheese, soft ripened 28
chewing 48
citrus fruits 59
coeliac disease 33
cow's milk 21–2, 30, 36, 58, 59
cups, using 57

dairy products 59
diet, healthy 12–13
dunkables 56–7

eggs 27

family meals 54, 58
fat 3, 6–7, 25
fatty foods 27
feeds:
    making up 24–5
    warming 24–5
Feingold, Dr Ben 36
fibre 7–8, 25, 27
finger-foods 48, 56–7
flavours, new 32, 51
follow-on milks 20–1
food allergies/intolerances
    32–3, 34–7
food fads 55
food safety 63–7
formula milk 20, 21
free-range foods 37–8
frozen foods 65
fussy eating 55–6

gluten intolerance 33
goat's milk 22

healthy eating 12–13
homemade foods 38–39,
    64–5, 67
hydrolysed vegetable protein
    27
hyperactivity 36–7

intolerances 32–3, 34–7
iron 11, 48–49

lumps 46

microwaves 49, 63–4
milk 14–22, 30, 31, 58
minerals 11–12
monosodium glutamate 28

non-starch polysaccharide
    (NSP) 7–8
nuts 28, 35

oats 28
organic foods 37–8

paté 27
peanuts, allergy to 34, 35
phenylketonuria 33–4
pre-term babies 32
proteins 3, 4–5
purées, freezing 67

readiness 31–2
recipes:
  apples:
    baked 141
    and kiwi yoghurt 117
    purée 73
  apricot, peach, nectarine
    and plum purée 83
  autumn pudding 120–1
  avocado:
    guacamole 139–40

and pear purée 84
purée 84
bananas:
  bake, with vanilla 142
  loaf 138–9
  purée 74
  rice with cinnamon 84
  smoothie 120
beans:
  baked beans and cheesy
    toast 102–3
  Caribbean rice 'n' peas
    135–7
  green bean purée 71
  kidney bean and tomato
    dinner 105
beef, spinach beef with
  tomato 128
bread and butter pudding
  with apricots 144–6
broccoli purée 72
bubble and squeak cakes
  106
butternut squash:
  and orange soup 88–9
  purée 69–70
Caribbean rice 'n' peas
  135–6
carrots:
  creamy carrots and
    parsnips with nutmeg
    76–8
  and parsnip soup 93
  purée 68
  soup with spinach and
    lentils 90–1
cauliflower:
  cheese 102
  purée 73
chappati 111
cheesy:
  dip, with mint, chives
    and cucumber 114–15
  fish shapes 134
  lentils with carrot 103
  muffins 112

potatoes and broccoli 110
cherries, special cherry
  and banana rice 81–3
chicken:
  banana and apple curry
    124–5
  Indian, with lime 123
  liver and apple casserole
    94
  with peaches and pasta
    94–5
  stock 85–6
  sweet and sour, with
    mango 123–4
cinnamon toast with
  mango 142
clapshot 80
corned beef hash 127
courgettes:
  lasagne 136–7
  purée 71
  risotto 109–10
couscous with courgette,
  pepper and mushrooms
  135
dried fruit purée 83–4
Eccles cakes 119–20
falafels 137–38
fish:
  chowder 133–4
  cooking methods 98
  with orange sauce 101
  pie with egg and tomato
    132–3
French toast 113
fruit salad, tropical 144
fruity:
  porridge 118
  white fish with cheese 99
Greek moussaka 129–30
guacamole 139–40
haddock:
  baked, with fennel and
    chives 99–100
  fish cakes with parsley
    and spring onions 101–2

hummus 140
Irish stew 89
kitcheri 107–09
lamb:
  meatballs with
    cinnamon, coconut and
    cardamom 128–9
  Moroccan, with beans
    130–1
  navarin of 97
lasagne, courgette 136–8
leek and potato soup 92
lentils, cheesy, with carrot
  103
mango:
  cream 115–16
  purée 82
meatballs, mini, with pasta
  shapes 131–3
meaty tomato, courgette
  and pasta 95–7
melon, mango and paw
  paw (papaya) purée 83
melon purée 82
minestrone 89–90
mixed root vegetable
  purée 77
moussaka 129–30
muesli 122–3
muffins, cheesy 112
omelette, veggie tortillas
  108
papaya purée 83
parsnips:
  creamed, with spinach
    79
  purée 69
pasta:
  with creamy leeks and
    tomato 104
  with tomato sauce 104–6
paw paw (papaya) purée
  83
peach melba 119
pear purée 73–4
peas:

creamy soup 92–4
green, purée 72
plaice with parsley and
chive sauce 100–1
polenta with oregano 114
porridge, fruity 118
potatoes:
baked, with cheesy
chives 103–4
with celeriac purée 81
cheesy, and broccoli 110
grated potato cakes with
chicken and vegetables
126
and pumpkin damper
111–12
purée 71
and swede purée 80
and watercress purée
79–80
pumpkin:
roasted, with cinnamon
78
and spinach purée 75–6
raspberry and passion
fruit sauce 143
rhubarb, stewed, with
orange custard 116
rice:
pudding 117
banana,
cinnamon and orange
143
fragrant, with
orange and cardamom
117–19
red, yellow and green
106–7
Thai coconut 141
rusks, homemade 113
shepherd's pie with
parsnip and potato mash
96–7
Singapore noodles with
chicken 125–6
snacks 145

spinach:
beef with tomato 128
purée with nutmeg 77
spring green purée 72
strawberry yoghurt,
homemade 119
swede purée 69
sweet pepper purée 78
sweet potatoes:
and carrot purée 79
and potato purée 79
purée 70
Thai coconut rice 141
toast:
cinnamon, with mango
142
French 113
tomatoes:
and cucumber raita 139
green bean and baby rice
dinner 76
rice with mushrooms
109
sauce 87
soup with basil 91
tortillas, veggie 108
tropical fruit salad 144
tuna broccoli bake 100
turnip purée 70
tzaziki 115
vegetable stock 86–7
veggie tortillas 108
white sauce 88
yoghurt, homemade
118–19
rice 67
rye 27

safety 63–4
salt (sodium chloride) 25–6
self-feeding 46–7
sheep's milk 22
smoked foods 27
snacks 58
soya milk 21, 36
spices 27

sterilization 23–4
sugar 5, 26, 66

tastes, introducing 31–2, 37
tea 28
teeth 45, 46
cleaning 51–2
protecting 51
teething 48
textures, new 32
toddlers 58

variety 45, 47
vegan diet 50
vegetarian diet 4–5, 49–50
vitamin C 10, 50
vitamins 8–11, 25
drops 46
preserving 64–5

water 8
weaning 30–44
weaning calendars:
four months 40–1
four-and-a-half months
42–3
five to six months 43–4
six to nine months 51–3
nine to twelve months
58–60
wheat 28
work, and breastfeeding
18–19